# unstable frontiers

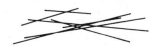

# unstable
## frontiers

**Technomedicine and the
Cultural Politics of "Curing" AIDS**

## john nguyet erni

 University of Minnesota Press
Minneapolis
London

Copyright 1994 by the Regents of the University of Minnesota

Part of this material has been previously published as "Articulating the (Im)possible: Popular Media and the Cultural Politics of 'Curing' AIDS," *Communication* 13 (1992): 39–56. Reprinted with permission of Gordon and Breach Science Publishers S.A.

Published by the University of Minnesota Press
2037 University Avenue Southeast, Minneapolis, MN 55455-3092
Printed in the United States of America on acid-free paper

Library of Congress Cataloging-in-Publication Data

Erni, John Nguyet.
   Unstable frontiers : technomedicine and the cultural politics of "curing"AIDS / John Nguyet Erni.
      p.   cm.
   Includes bibliographical references and index.
   ISBN 0-8166-2380-5 (acid-free paper). —ISBN 0-8166-2381-3 (pbk. : acid-free paper)
   1. AIDS (Disease)—Social aspects.   2. AIDS (Disease) in mass media.   I. Title.
RA644.A25E76   1994
362.1'969792—dc20                                                                94-773
                                                                                   CIP

The University of Minnesota is an
equal-opportunity educator and employer.

To my loving father
Elias Rosano Erni,
1930–1990

# Contents

# Acknowledgments

Like many other works on AIDS, this book grew out of anger and sorrow. It also came out of several turbulent years of trying to develop my own foreign identity and voice in the American professional academic environment and in the gay social world. In this process, I learned how to unlearn an epidemic.

Lawrence Grossberg blessed me with his brilliance, encouragement, friendship, integrity, sense of humor, and inspiring criticisms throughout the writing of this book, and throughout a journey that has only begun. He is the best mentor in the world.

I am also deeply grateful to Paula Treichler's assistance and critical commentary, particularly during the research phase of this book. Many warm thanks also go to Lisa Cartwright, Norman Denzin, James Hay, Kevin Kopelson, and Cindy Patton, all of whom pushed me for clarity and strength in my arguments.

My editor, Janaki Bakhle, has been instrumental in making this book possible. I want to thank her for believing in the work of a young scholar and for giving me strength in ways she may not realize. Roberta Hughey and Laura Westlund offered their excellent assistance in matters of accuracy, precision, and clarity in my expression of ideas. This book benefited greatly from their help. Thanks especially to Robert Mosimann for extending all kinds of technical assistance necessary for publication. Being extremely organized and sane at the same time, Robert possesses a rare combination of qualities that I envy.

My dear friend Terry Brown has been a great confidant and partner during the past four years. I learned from her how to live and work with integrity in my scholarship and passion in my teaching. I admire her reflective soul.

Many more friends and colleagues have provided me with support, patience, insight, fun conversations, and love, including Anne Balsamo, Christopher Boudewyn, Douglas Crimp, Ann Darling, Larry Harred, James W. Pratt, and the folks at the University of Wisconsin–River Falls.

I wish my father had lived to read this book. For a while, things were very unfair to him.

# Introduction

In *Unstable Frontiers*, I explore the cultural politics that arises from the question of medical treatment in the AIDS crisis. I propose that the current powerful scientific and commercial project of "searching for a cure for AIDS"—a label that has become a master code in the language used to describe AIDS treatment developments in the scientific and popular arenas—is structured by the contradictory but stable definitions of AIDS as being at the same time curable and incurable. This underlying binary discourse of curability/incurability frames the way we conceptualize and struggle with the issues of medical treatment for AIDS. I argue that an understanding of AIDS treatment, and more broadly an understanding of the politics of "technomedicine"—broadly defined as technologically oriented, commercially structured, regulatory medicine—at this historical juncture must incorporate a critical analysis of this discourse. And I assume that the useful starting place for that critical analysis is the theory of discourse developed in Michel Foucault's work and the theory of articulation developed in British cultural studies.

In this book, I do not see the work of "curing AIDS" as merely a fact of biomedical research, endowed with the technoethics and energies typically associated with a scientific endeavor. Any AIDS scientist can provide a narrative of that kind. Nor do I attempt to offer "practical" guidelines about treatment options. Detailed compilations of such guidelines and brilliant analyses of the practical utilities of treatment information have been provided, vigilantly and persistently, by AIDS activist organizations and their community-based publications, such as John James's *AIDS Treatment News*, *Treatment Issues* of the Gay Men's Health Crisis, Project Inform's *PI Perspective*, *PWA Coalition Newsline* from the People with AIDS Coalition, and many other regional publications. Yet this book would not have been possible without the social commitment, technical competence, and practical insight of AIDS activists and scientists; in their own historical and structural contexts, they have shaped, in similar or contradictory ways, the terrain of discourse regarding "curing AIDS" to which my analysis is directed.

Specifically, this book is concerned with "curing AIDS" as a cultural and political phenomenon constituted by a set of discursive practices and representations that determine the complex realities of AIDS treatment, including the structure of the phenomenon and what legitimates it; the network of technologies, procedures, apparatuses, and actions that arise as possibilities (and impossibilities) within that structure; the cultural narratives that represent it; the cultural fantasies that sustain and perpetuate it; and the wider historical conjuncture from which it appears and within which it is transformed. From media journalism, including television and press coverage, news in the alternative press, popular magazines, special documentary programs, television talk shows, and community newsletters created by AIDS organizations, come the textual materials that shape the way we grasp and come to terms with the biomedical response to AIDS. All this is part of the phenomenon of "curing AIDS." It is within this discursive trajectory, and not only in the research laboratory, that a technoethical consciousness about AIDS treatment has emerged, through which the politics of the control of the medicalized body is shaped.

An underlying assumption of this book is that the "cure" inscribes highly specific languages, embodies particular historical and institutional structures, directs a network of technological practices, and excites deep-rooted popular cultural fantasies about the human body in illness; in short, it is a discourse. An analysis of the overall project of curing AIDS cannot be carried out without identifying such languages, structures, practices, and fantasies by which the project itself is created. The realities of medical treatment cannot be imagined as an ontological matter to which discourse refers; no process or practice lies outside detailed discursive systems. To be sure, "curing AIDS" is an object of knowledge made possible on the one hand by the network of techniques and rational programmatic procedures of modern technomedicine, and on the other hand by representational codes, statements, narratives, and images appearing in medical journals and the media. Once we see that the project of "curing AIDS" is inaugurated as a historically specific discursive knowledge, we may begin to examine the power relations that inhere in it. There are mortal stakes under the sign of "curing AIDS."

Because in many ways our mortal hopes for surviving HIV/AIDS, which bear a *constructed* relationship to the designated status of "being cured," turn on revisioning the world as discourse with which we must learn to live, I want to discuss the important relation of discourse to "reality." Consider, for instance, the ubiquitous "fact" that "AIDS is incurable" and the varying degree of visibility of its discursive dimensions as expressed in the following statements:

1. There is no cure for AIDS.

2. The Annual International Conference on AIDS, which has been dominated by Western professional medicine, has declared that to date there is no cure for AIDS.

3. The mainstream medical establishment declares that no antiviral drug or vaccine, or any combination of such therapeutic means, has successfully disrupted or halted the growth of the human immunodeficiency virus (HIV) or eradicated it entirely from the human body. HIV, an acronym adopted in 1986 by the international scientific community, is hypothesized as the cause of AIDS, and thereby is the target for a cure.

4. In the United States, the national medical institutions have declared that HIV/AIDS is incurable. Epidemiology has declared that no infected persons have successfully been able to rid themselves of HIV. HIV testing, which is designed to detect the existence of HIV antibodies, has declared that no infected persons have been able to reverse their serostatus. Clinical medicine has declared that the symptoms in all infected individuals express a linear, progressive, and multiplying development. Immunology has declared that the immune systems of all infected individuals experience a steady downward decline. Virology and molecular genetics have declared that HIV mutates in unexplainable ways and could undermine or reverse any therapeutic advances made by existing approved antiviral drugs such as azidothymidine (AZT), dideoxyinosine (ddI), or dideoxycytidine (ddC). Prophylactic or preventive medicine has declared that, although it may be able to stave off the onset of symptoms temporarily, it cannot eliminate HIV. All of these declarations are made in the assumption that no scientific study conducted in Western medicine has yet offered any necessary and sufficient counterproof.

5. The set of historically developed and adopted technomedical practices employed to study AIDS has declared that an eradication of HIV is extremely difficult to achieve. Virological, molecular, and genetic studies of HIV's behavior, life cycle, and points of vulnerability have supported this premise. Clinical trials of experimental drugs, the key method for developing treatments for diseases during the past sixty years in the United States and one supported by legislatures and commercial pharmaceutical ventures in a competitive market environment, have shown that no compound can yet eradicate HIV from the human body. Clinical trials are three phased, randomized, double blinded, and placebo controlled, conducted by scientific and university centers overseen by the Food and Drug Administration (FDA). Their validity is measured by such accepted

scientific standards as "proof of safety and efficacy" and the use of "pure controlled subjects." This highly controlled set of methodical practices is hypothesized to be the best way to develop drugs for AIDS.

6. Alternative healing practices provided by community institutions outside of, and peripheral to, the structure of the national medical establishment, which have employed a combination of Western and non-Western medicine ranging from acupuncture to herbal treatments and which have developed their own institutional forms (for example, buyers' clubs), are largely considered "unscientific" and are therefore not accepted as viable curing practices for AIDS. Meanwhile, alternative theories of AIDS, which have significantly challenged the scientific validity of the HIV model (e.g., see Root-Bernstein, 1993) and which have proposed alternative methods to develop treatment for AIDS, have only begun to surface in mainstream scientific discussions.

This exercise[1] illustrates how a widely accepted "fact"—that is, statement 1—arises from a whole discursive machine (the fact being the tip of a discursive pyramid) that, through adding different linguistic markers indicating histories, agents, disciplines, and social formations, contextualizes the fact in specific provinces of meanings that have arisen from social and historical institutions and from a specific network of material practices, procedures, methods, and so on. Such a discursive context also acquires its validity by marginalizing other beliefs contextualized by other institutions, histories, agents, and practices. In this way, scientific discourse is magic, for, in Paula Treichler's words, it is "a form of shorthand in which facts, once admitted, need no longer retain the history of their fabrication" (1992a, p. 86).

As the statements in this exercise unfold from the apodictic statement 1 to the highly contextualized statements that follow, however, we witness an emergence of a "medical paradigm" enacted around the scientific development of the "AIDS cure." This paradigm is unique in that (1) it is largely a Western medical perspective; (2) it is an expression of the underlying, rarely disputed HIV model and therefore subscribes to the "magic bullet" model of treatment development; and (3) it is subjected to change based on conflicting social and political needs and demands.

When this medical paradigm suggesting the incurability of AIDS reaches the popular arena primarily through the mass media, the statement "There is no cure for AIDS" can and has been translated into such free-floating but powerful statements as "AIDS is deadly," "AIDS is invariably fatal," and "HIV seropositivity means a guaranteed death sentence." This fatalistic view generates a linguistic baggage that marks people as "AIDS victims" infected by the "AIDS virus," who are to be separated from the "general public." This linguistic baggage turns on cultural fantasies about the body, its sexuality (homosexuality in particular), morbidity, and temporality in relation to the imagined status of being "cured."

Just as this whole discursive machine by which the incurability of AIDS gets constructed is trundled out onto the field, it is met with an equally complex discourse that has also appeared as a "fact" or a "claim": "A cure for AIDS is possible in time." Hence we witness a wholly different economy—histories, institutions, agents, practices, popular beliefs, and cultural fantasies—underlying this "fact." We also observe that the interface of the two discourses, with its contradiction and tension as well as conjoinment and articulation, creates a spectacular sociopsychological drama that continues to affect our practical struggles over AIDS treatment issues. In a culture's imagination, the "cure," like the HIV, being both fact and fabrication, becomes a reality that is too risky and too costly to give up. To the degree that the "cure" is both factual and fabricated, there are real stakes in living (and dying) under the pervasive signs of "There is no cure for AIDS" and "A cure for AIDS is possible in time."

In this way, discourse is anything but disembodied or decontextualized. It is precisely at the acute point of the real that discourses live, mutate, die, or get resurrected. A discourse, far from being a matter of arbitrarily creating reality in its own image (as some may say), is a matter of a sharply unarbitrary engagement with reality. The body, far from being "abandoned" after discourse, is the very flesh of it, because unless the dynamic processes of representations and practices cease to appear to speak the "truth" of the body, the material body itself will always remain the generator for discourse.

In this book, the questions that I discuss are not those arguing for or against technomedicine, although my strongest motive is to challenge technomedicine's response to the crisis. Rather, the questions that seem most culturally and politically charged are internal to technomedicine. The core chapters of this book discuss such internal contradictions. The contradictions, I argue, arise from the overall, totalizing perspective of the curability/incurability of AIDS.

There are three such contradictions. The first is the pervasive contradiction between the tendency to promote medical innovations as the triumph of science and the tendency to undermine such innovations, vigilantly calling attention to science's own limitations. Reports of potential AIDS treatment are frequently fractured around this contradiction. Chapter 1 explores this contradiction, using AZT as a case study. The second contradiction lies in seeing AIDS on the one hand as a newly evolved pathological condition that, "by nature," eludes scientific understanding and on the other hand as a biotechnical matter that can be reasonably discerned, if not confidently mastered and penetrated, by modern technological medicine. Chapter 2 argues that this contradiction is the main structuring principle of the entire question of AIDS treatment. The third contradiction involves imagining HIV infection as a process with an internal, largely hidden, self-regulating mechanism that determines its own temporal course of infectivity versus seeing HIV infection as a process upon which an external, technically and institutionally constructed regulatory system can be imposed that can control but not alter its course. Virological medicine tends to support the former view, while clinical research tends to support the latter. I argue that this contradiction lies in the divergent cultural imaginations of the temporal logic of HIV infection. In chapter 3 I demonstrate that temporality is a very important dimension in the cultural narratives of "curing AIDS," constituting a peculiar structural logic in the AIDS treatment discourse. Time has also been the central point of struggle between the AIDS activists and the Food and Drug Administration. In fact, the construction of a whole temporal consciousness around AIDS has served to legitimize a powerful definition—indeed, restriction—of the "proper" method for developing treatment for AIDS.

The discursive field of "curing AIDS" is studded with contradictions: between the rhetoric of high hopes and cautionary skepticism, between the power of modern technological medicine and the hidden, menacing power of a "new" pathology, between different temporalized clusters of medical knowledge. Contradictions do not always imply conflicts, however. An important argument of this book is that contradictions are an essential part of a discourse that is trying to gain control of the devastating crisis. In fact, contradictions can be harnessed, reified, and regulated on a mass scale for a powerful enforcement around curing/controlling. The social power that the attention to curing generates rests less on its command of unity/stability than on its deployment of contradiction/instability. Such a proliferation of contradictions/instabilities—the "unstable frontiers" of AIDS—creates an economy that can be at once phantasmic and paranoid. The complex drama of stability/instability is the crucial carrier of political power.

Seen in this way, the perpetual sense of crisis-uncertainty-contradiction in the AIDS treatment discourse is not so much a threat to the existing structure of society and technomedicine; it may in fact be the willful tool of power. The formation of the discourse of "curing AIDS" therefore requires setting the terms of, and profiting from, the perpetual sense of crisis, always dissolving into a massive anxiety provoked by a paradox: the definition of the curability/incurability of AIDS.

In the broader historical conjuncture, these contradictions reveal some larger transformations of technomedicine with respect to its historical crisis of authority. They also inscribe new "subjects of curing" within science, of course, but also within the AIDS treatment activist movement. In science, as in the activist movement, the subjects of curing have been acutely connected with the shifting "gay subjectivity" (particularly the gay male subject) and queer politics. In this way, technomedicine's struggle over its historical crisis of authority cannot be thought of separately from the shifting formations of gay subjectivity. Chapter 4 is devoted to examining these conjunctural effects.

Chapter 5 retraces the theoretical trajectory implicitly covered in the earlier chapters, placing "curing AIDS" explicitly within the framework of a theory of discourse and a theory of articulation. It also provides an overview of the cultural criticisms aimed at analyzing the media's representations of AIDS, which will help to clarify the form of critique of the media that I undertake in this book.

It is important to determine the periodization for this study. The construct "curing AIDS" did not enter the popular lexicon until the second half of the 1980s. The early years of the epidemic, it has been widely recognized, were characterized by a media blackout and widespread panic. AIDS treatment research began during those years but was largely hidden from public consciousness. An important break in the received history of the epidemic came in 1987: the antiviral drug AZT was "invented" and approved for public use, giving rise, in my view, to the birth or integration of an emerging consciousness about "curing AIDS." I therefore arbitrarily take this point, the first quarter of 1987, to be the beginning of the period for this project.

Over the next few years, massive press coverage of new developments of drug and vaccine research appeared. During this period, a large body of reports and commentaries from journalists, scientists, experts, health-care professionals, representatives of drug companies, representatives of AIDS community organizations, and AIDS activists began to flow into all sectors of public discussion, deepening society's conviction—and confusion—about a titanic crusade full of moralistic, political, and historical implications. At this point, old standards were challenged and new visions were introduced, traditional organizational strategies were forced to undergo reassessment, "business-as-usual" modes of operations were highly politicized, and community collaborative initiatives were quickly and efficiently organized (see Epstein, 1991; Finkelstein, 1990; Edgar and Rothman, 1991, 1992; Treatment Action Group, 1992). By the late 1980s, an accumulated set of concerns regarding AIDS treatment was set in steady motion, complete with a series of historical dramas, a plethora of themes and ideologies, and a handful of highly visible agencies and individuals who were the key players in the AIDS treatment discourse.

Two moments during this time are particularly noteworthy. During the Sixth International Conference on AIDS held in San Francisco in the summer of 1990, new findings for the possibilities of combination antiviral drug and vaccine treatments were reported, signaling a renewed optimism over the prospect of AIDS treatment. With the adoption of new procedures, there seemed to be a turning point in the reconceptualization of the whole paradigm of clinical drug trials. In contrast, at the Eighth International Conference on AIDS in Amsterdam in the summer of 1992, it was reported that the progress of combination therapy research and vaccine research was only incremental. The most troubling news concerned HIV's ability to mutate its own genetic structure, an ability that threatened to undermine the knowledge about the virus gained in the past years. A looming pessimism surrounding the conference was quickly echoed in the popular arena. In order to include these significant markers in the history of AIDS treatment research in my analysis, I have chosen the summer of 1992, again arbitrarily, as the closing point of my analysis.

To become familiar with the central players and events related to the treatment issues of AIDS, the reader may consult the Appendix, which outlines the major treatment-related events as they were covered by network television news within the period of this study (January 1987-June 1992). The first reports of AIDS treatment activities and controversies, however, began in 1985, so I have included the pre-AZT treatment activities in the Appendix.

# 1 Paralysis or Breakthrough: The Making and Unmaking of AZT

> The challenge is learning how and when to use it, and how and when to stop using it.
>
> Project Inform, fact sheet on AZT, 1988

> But the debate about AZT, like AIDS treatment activism in general, is inevitably about the uses and consequences of technology and biomedical theory in everyday life. Hence it is a debate, with mortal stakes, about the evolution, value, and possible limits of a radically democratic technoculture.
>
> Paula A. Treichler, "How to Have a Theory in an Epidemic"

> If we wrapped the drug [AZT] in a £10 note and gave it away, people would say it cost too much.
>
> Alfred Shepperd, recently retired chairman of Wellcome PLC, Burroughs Wellcome's British parent

> Says Uwe E. Reinhardt, a Princeton economist specializing in health care: "Clever drug companies stick their research overhead on a patient group that won't complain. You pluck the goose that squeals the least." Burroughs, he says, "plucked the wrong goose."
>
> Brian O'Reilly, "The Inside Story of the AIDS Drug"

Medical breakthroughs are jealously guarded social assets. Situated between hope, competition, doubt, and even cynicism, they carry a peculiar kind of authority: on the one hand, they may proclaim the triumph of science and medicine, and on the other, they have the power to generate confusion and ambiguous expectations. Although the idea of a "breakthrough" commonly delineates originality, newness, progress, and success, the social commentary about a medical breakthrough—created especially by the medical community and echoed in the media—often tells a different story. Its proclamation is almost always accompanied by words of skepticism, contained in a caution against false expectation that seeks to prevent undue public reaction and at the same time creates a perplexity—indeed, a discourse of impasse—over what really to make of the breakthrough news. The story about the discovery of AZT found in the news exemplifies, exactly, the construction of such an impasse.

1

Hailed as a medical breakthrough, AZT, the only approved antiviral treatment for AIDS until 1990, once awed the press and the public, tendered new hope for AIDS patients, and sparked new prospects for treatment development among medical researchers. Yet, from the outset, conflicting theories and experiences of the drug created continual debate over its usefulness. As a result, interlaboratory competition was intensified, and many patients felt profound confusion over whether this drug would benefit them. The debate over AZT's usefulness goes on, even though the drug has been approved for wide market distribution since 1987. The press, I shall argue, has contributed to the confusion.

Medical explanations of the drug by researchers alone do little to explain its social and political effects. Nor do they address the power structure from which the drug is created. That AZT is not only a medical discovery but also a social and political phenomenon has at least three possible implications:

1. AZT rekindles a strong sentiment of scientific triumph over diseases, sparking an overall sense of rejuvenation of the social and cultural authority of medical sciences. This authority has its conceptual roots in the modern postwar paradigm of medical treatment in terms of antibiotic intervention, commonly known as the "magic bullet" model of curing diseases.

2. The medical paradigm that guides the development of AZT—that is, a model of treatment grounded in the intervention at a specific point in the life cycle of a single agent known as HIV—has dominated subsequent drug research for AIDS. AZT has become a model drug that shapes the priority, structure, and direction of mainstream AIDS treatment research.

3. Although treating AIDS is generally recognized as a complex matter involving more than drug treatment, the media and medical discourses about AIDS treatment continue to feature AZT at its center. The discovery of AZT created the first sign that the epidemic was "under control," yet it emerged from a contradictory climate of doubts over AZT's status as a "cure." On the one hand, the drug has profoundly shaped our imagination of the possibility for an AIDS treatment, but on the other hand AZT has an ambivalent relation to "curing" in the overall language of treatment. In fact, it produces an overwhelming sense of uncertainty regarding AIDS treatment as a whole. The debate over

AZT's efficacy as a drug cannot be thought of separately from how the drug is represented.

An emphasis on AZT may obscure the fact that multiple AIDS treatment options exist, many of which are much less costly or toxic.[1] While we must demand a diversity of protocols and designs for testing drugs, a recognition of the potential usefulness of multiple alternative treatment options, and a reduction of repetitive AZT trials, we must also examine the important ways in which the AZT story has structured the entire narrative about "curing AIDS."[2] In order to challenge the discursive centrism of AZT, we must begin by identifying the knowledges, representations, and effects articulated by its story.

In this chapter, I analyze how the discovery of AZT arose from a highly specific—and narrow—paradigm that informed mainstream biomedicine's treatment research, and how this paradigm has been perpetuated in subsequent research. The emergence of the AZT model, we now realize, has significantly limited intervention options for treating AIDS. Yet, this particular model has its conceptual—and therefore political and economic—roots in the modern postwar medical paradigm.

I then construct a chronological and media history of AZT. Particular attention will be paid to the social preconditions and narrative themes that structure the AZT phenomenon. The "official" and media histories of the drug weave together a field of discourse underscored by deep-seated contradictions and tensions. Such contradictions and tensions not only encapsulate the real puzzlement over AZT's usefulness as a treatment, they seem to *valorize* the modern medical paradigm that informs the scientific "discovery" of the drug itself. The AZT story revealed in this reconstructed history appears to be an unstable narrative, however; it seems caught in the increasingly unstable dominance of the same medical paradigm that it valorizes.

The analysis of the scientific paradigm that structures the making of AZT and the analysis of the social and media history of the drug will lay the foundation for a mode of criticism used in this book. This criticism focuses on how the collusion of scientific, media, and public health policy discourses produce contradictory narratives about the reality of AIDS treatment within a particular shifting historical conjuncture.

The analysis presented in this chapter will open and close with a brief critique of an exemplary media representation of AZT. The first example appears to account comprehensively for the development of AIDS drugs, and particularly for the discovery of AZT, and the second example appears as a response to the government's announcement in the summer of 1989 that AZT could be beneficial to the asymptomatic HIV-infected population. I use these exemplary reports to examine how they help to transform AZT into a structural force that has promoted certain kinds of thought patterns and enabled a certain political agenda, and prohibited other kinds of thought patterns and agendas. This chapter attempts to explore this structuration process and its cultural and political implications, both in terms of how the AZT story is constructed and how it is embedded in the broader historical conjuncture.

## AZT in the Media (I): "Discovering" AZT

In what specific sense is AZT considered a "success story"? How has it been celebrated as a scientific triumph as well as a social blessing? The feature article "Where Are the Drugs to Cure AIDS?" that appeared in the *Chicago Tribune Magazine* on September 25, 1988, is one typical story about AZT's success as a treatment as well as a cultural symbol of medical authority.

Feature stories signify a movement away from the foreground (event, issue, dilemma) to the background (cause, motivation, explanation) of a problem, a news process that draws on a wide ideological field (see Hall et al., 1978). By assembling the elements of the background—people, places, experiences—the feature contextualizes the event, marking the parameter of the background problem and connecting the media process-es with more widely distributed popular ideologies. The *Tribune* feature article does exactly that. It does not simply represent a local interpreta-tion of the AIDS drug development process; it also serves to distill a larg-er cultural narrative about "rational medicine" by mobilizing a cultural memory of past medical conquests, bringing back the authority of medi-cine through the AZT story.

Both the narrative structure and the central themes developed in the *Tribune* story help to locate AZT at its center. Using a straightforward enigma/enigma-solving narrative structure, the story assembles a string of histories, institutions, and people to culminate in a rather authoritative explanation of the development and impact of AZT. Most noticeable are three subnarratives that are invoked as important "memory markers" of modern medicine.

The first, which appears as a lead-in to the article, summons a testimony of a woman named Anne Miller, who, after a miscarriage in 1942, suffered blood poisoning that almost killed her. Her physician, Dr. Orvan Hess, "a pioneering Yale obstetrician," decided to try an experimental drug that had been studied for fourteen years—penicillin. The narrative proceeds with a suspenseful description of how the drug performed a miracle and saved Miller's life. Hess is depicted as a young fellow who tried to convince older physicians at a medical meeting about the wonder of penicillin and was "politely" brushed aside. The narrative connects a historical description of the event with reflective comments by both Miller and Hess thirty-five years later. It concludes:

> On that fateful morning in New Haven when Anne Miller's temperature dropped to normal after her near-fatal miscarriage, there was born in America the art and science of modern drug development. The advent of penicillin and the other antibiotics seemed like such a fairy tale that modern drug development was born with a sense of great expectations. (Breo, p. 12)

We are offered here a history lesson, woven together by the images of a courageous physician, a thankful patient, and a miracle cure—a lesson about the rise of modern medicine as a force for salvation.

The second story recalls Dr. Otis Owen, the former secretary of the Department of Health and Human Services, and his experience with experimental drugs. Described as someone who "knows the frustration of having nothing to offer patients who are desperately ill and are in excruciating pain," Owen was determined to find some relief for his wife, who was suffering from multiple myeloma in 1981. The drugs DMSO (dimethysulfoxide) and THC (tetrahydrocannabinol) were the most effective painkillers he could locate, but neither was approved for human use: one was a drug to treat horses, and the other was an active ingredient of marijuana. His wife eventually died. Owen lamented, "Why can't a dying person, with severe pain, have easy prescription access to helpful medication?" Following Owen's story is a counternarrative about the exorbitant number of prescriptions filled in this country. It cites a string of figures to show how drug firms have flooded the market with excessive "me too" formulations, especially cold and cough preparations. The story leads to a description of how the FDA effectively eliminated many useless drugs from the market.

If the first story conjures history, the second bespeaks motives. It suggests that the motive of making experimental drugs available for patients with severe conditions must be balanced with the motive of rationally controlling unnecessary prescriptions. This story thus begins to articulate one of the chief themes in the world of AIDS cure discourse: rational balance.

A mother's struggle to help find a cure for her children's affliction is the third story in the report leading to the nucleus AZT story. In 1977, Abbey Myers's children all suffered from Tourette syndrome. The report recites her painful description of her children's bizarre, involuntary physical and vocal tics and of how Pimozide, the only experimental drug thought to be useful at the time, was blocked by the FDA because of insufficient trial data that proved its efficacy. Frustrated, Myers contacted the FDA but was rudely dismissed. She later joined the Tourette Society as a volunteer and began a crusade that led to the establishment of the Orphan Drug Act of 1983.[3] The narrative concludes with Myers's happy account of the recovery of all her children.

Tucked between these three subnarratives is a brief historical account of the development of the FDA. Central to this interlude is an emphasis on three specific moments of the FDA's history: the cases of Elixir Sulfanilamide and Thalidomide, and the establishment of the Treatment Investigational New Drug (IND) Amendment.[4] The first two moments are used to underscore the acquisition of the FDA's power in setting the "standards of strength and purity" (p. 12). In virtually every media discussion of the history of the FDA, the case of Thalidomide is invoked as a central narrative component for validating the administration's regulatory power. The moment of the establishment of the Treatment IND Amendment is invoked as the FDA's reformist gesture in a time of crisis. All of this is part of the AZT discourse.

The schematic mobilization of articulators—ideological conductors—structures how AZT is going to be understood. The articulators in this case are, in thematic terms:

1. The courage of the physician to go against the grain of current medical beliefs;
2. The rational balance between individual and public medical needs;
3. The image of an individual's crusade in fighting bureaucracy;
4. The image of the government as a protector of general interest and as a reformer during critical times (centered on the FDA).

Corollary themes include the woman as victim, the rareness and severity of the disease, human suffering and death, and the random success of drugs. All of this articulates the historical and structural arena within which the happy discovery of AZT emerged.

In the report, the AZT story that follows the three subnarratives has, in a real sense, already been told. At its center is Dr. Sam Broder of the National Cancer Institute, who, described as taking a different position from other scientists at the time of AZT's initial trials, explains:

> When it comes to predictions about drug development, I believe that the pessimists have a worse track record than the optimists. I believe in science, and I believe that in this line of work you have to be an optimist. . . . Our research patients are courageous pioneers, and our young lab scientists are taking tremendous intellectual and physical risks in working with live AIDS virus. (p. 18)

Indeed a Dr. Hess of the 1980s, Broder is willing to try anything. The report continues by citing his view of the importance of federal government-supported science in the development of AZT, and then recites the process of AZT's discovery in order to emphasize how the Treatment IND Amendment benefited the process by which AZT was approved. "AZT is a formal validation of the science of drug development and the perfect example of the need for carefully controlled clinical trials," proclaims Broder (cited in Breo, p. 20).

Far from being an individual medical discovery, AZT arises from and eventually feeds back into a larger network of historical narratives and memories. Now AZT bears a history *outside* this current epidemic, a historical connection that the *Tribune* report ideologically affirms.

In a 1990 press release, "The Age of Antivirals: A New Era in Medicine," Burroughs Wellcome, the pharmaceutical company that discovered and manufactures AZT, claims that viruses are the new "formidable enemy" of drug researchers, constituting a new era of medical science. The success of penicillin as an antibacterial agent is again cited, the struggle of individual researchers making bold steps in viral research again invoked. Rational, controlled design is the preferred approach to drug discovery:

> The search for . . . targets [for attack] and development of new strategies is the story of antiviral research, and the search begins with a new idea for drug discovery—the rational approach. Rather than randomly screen for useful activity, the rational approach attempts to design a compound that will act in a specific way. (p. 4)

The report goes on to describe the company's history of viral research in the past decades, following this rational approach. The discovery of

AZT, therefore, arises from this history in this new age of medical science: "With . . . extensive experience in antiviral research, it was natural for Burroughs Wellcome to be at the forefront of the effort to find a treatment for HIV-infection" (p. 11). Aside from the obvious rhetoric of self-advertisement in this press release, the report constructs a broad, historical terrain—"The Age of Antivirals"—within which one (narrow) mode of medical intervention into infectious diseases (i.e., antiviral treatment) is endorsed and preferred. A chain of discursive connections has been forged: viruses mark a new research focus, antiviral research marks a new medical era, and Burroughs Wellcome marks an appropriate corporate research response. Thus, we see the heavily emphasized significance of AZT not so much as a product of technomedicine as a product of its "natural history." Here I am concerned not with the scientific validity of antiviral research, so much as with its ideology, the possibilities it promotes, and the options it prohibits. HIV infection causes immunocompromise; treatment clearly requires more than an interruption of the virus's life cycle by an antiviral agent. Ultimately, treatment requires a conception that goes beyond an antiviral attack. This brings into focus the fundamental question about the sort of scientific vision that holds the validity of the AZT discovery together.

## The AZT Paradigm

Central to the creation of AIDS treatment from the scientific point of view is the image of the life cycle of HIV. The key strategy—indeed, the underlying philosophy—of AIDS treatment is envisioned as a systematic attack on the virus's life span. The specific stages of the virus's replicating mechanism become the specific targets for attack. This makes the theory of a "rational" approach to drug development possible. Scientists themselves speak of "customized antibodies" that could be designed to act as a "bloodhound-and-policeman team" that "sniffs out [the activities of] the virus" and activates the immune system into destroying the virus (Yarchoan et al., 1988, p. 114). Recurrent words such as "blocking," "inhibiting," and "arresting" frame the language of strategies for intervention into the virus's life journey (see fig. 1).The underpinning conceptualization of control thus lies in a rational masterminding of the enemy's points of vulnerability.

In the scientific report by Yarchoan and his colleagues, the creation of AZT emerges from the explanation of the viral life previously described.

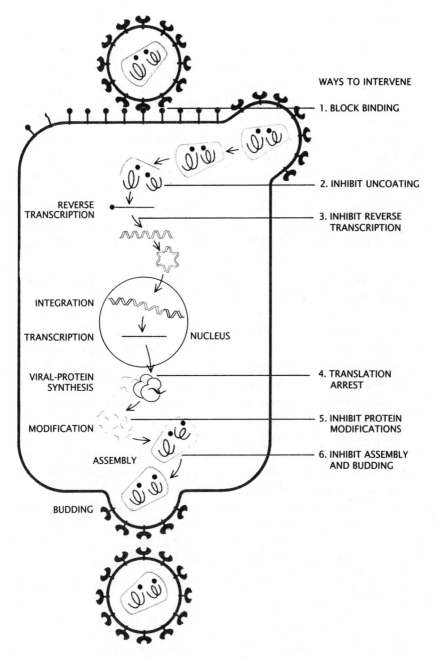

WAYS TO INTERVENE

1. BLOCK BINDING

2. INHIBIT UNCOATING

REVERSE
TRANSCRIPTION

3. INHIBIT REVERSE
TRANSCRIPTION

INTEGRATION

TRANSCRIPTION          NUCLEUS

VIRAL-PROTEIN
SYNTHESIS

4. TRANSLATION
ARREST

MODIFICATION

5. INHIBIT PROTEIN
MODIFICATIONS

ASSEMBLY

6. INHIBIT ASSEMBLY
AND BUDDING

BUDDING

Figure 1. HIV and a scientific structure of knowledge. Treatment is a strategic master-minding of the enemy's vulnerability. Illustration by Hans Iken from "AIDS Therapies," by Robert Yarchoan, Hiroaki Mitsuya, and Samuel Broder; copyright 1988 by Scientific American, Inc. All rights reserved.

The drug AZT works something like this. AZT interrupts and halts the genetic conversion process (from RNA to DNA) activated by the enzyme reverse transcriptase, a process deemed essential to the unique character of HIV. The power of AZT lies in its ability to attack the key step of HIV replication. Strictly speaking, however, AZT does not attack HIV. Because it resembles the genetic materials (nucleotides) that serve as building blocks in DNA and RNA, AZT masquerades its way to a false binding with the enzyme (reverse transcriptase) in the genetic conversion process.[5] This is a process of "competitive inhibition"—competitive because it strives to displace the nucleotides that ordinarily bind with the enzyme. After the binding, because AZT does not possess the necessary chemical group [hydroxyl (OH) group] that enables the genetic chain to continue, HIV's replication is forced to a stop. This is known as chain termination. A structure of knowledge emerges from this science of treatment that can be charted systematically (see table 1).

A scientific and circular logic is thus achieved: microbiological understanding of the virus justifies a need for "designer" drugs that reciprocally legitimize microbiological knowledge as the key "truth" necessary for effective intervention into the disease. In many crucial ways, AZT validates and perpetuates this whole structure of scientific knowledge; it serves as an interlocutor who holds the entire scientific vision together.

Arguably, the core of mainstream scientific research for AIDS treatment to date extends from this singular view, which reduces treatment to basic, microbiological research (a view that predates AIDS). A set of medical arguments and practices now supports it, particularly those that support the controlled placebo-trials method. Alternative, unorthodox forms of therapy not founded on microbiological research are thus structurally subordinated to this dominant view. The primary objection here is not to basic or microbiology research itself so much as to the critically limited research paradigm that has mostly been engineered around the AZT model. Activist Mark Harrington explains:

> People with AIDS have different priorities. Finding a "magic bullet" against HIV is a daunting task; some experts believe it is impossible. By contrast, secondary AIDS infections can quickly be made treatable. . . . It is not a question of ignoring antivirals, but of striking the right balance. This the ACTG [AIDS Clinical Trials Group] has not done. (1990, p. 40)

Harrington goes on to state that 80 percent of all the studies conducted by ACTG are studies of AZT, even though the drug has been on the mar-

## Table I. The AZT paradigm

| Postulation | Implication | Reasoned Action |
| --- | --- | --- |
| 1. A theory of a single infecting agent | A unified enigma | Microbiological intervention—the antibiotic treatment model—as the heart of treatment |
| 2. A discrete chartable course of infection | Distinguishable vulnerable points | Customized attack corresponding to vulnerable points |
| 3. A structural genetic resemblance | An illusion of authenticity as competitive advantage | Location of compounds that bear the resemblance |

ket since 1987. By May 1990, only one-sixth of the ACTG trials tested drugs against secondary infections and cancer.

Very little is new about medical science's reduction of treatment to research. In many ways, the AZT story merely retraces the success story of penicillin as an antibacterial drug at a time when bacterial germs were the unified enigma for medical scientists. In fact, the centrality given to penicillin as *the* model for modern medical therapy can be traced back to the celebrated discovery of Salvarsan by Paul Ehrlich in 1910 (Brandt, 1987, pp. 161-82). The insistence by scientists such as Robert Gallo and many others that AIDS can be explained by a unified enigma centered in HIV, despite conflicting views expressed by other similarly credible scientists (see, for example, Root-Bernstein, 1993), appears to resolve the whole question about the "cause" of AIDS and thus forges a focus for scientific research. The HIV theory, it has now been recognized, commands the entire field of AIDS treatment research, based on the magic-bullet model already mentioned. AZT—indeed the reemergence and domination of antiviral research in AIDS science as a whole—is anchored upon this historical paradigm.

From the outset, the media have assisted in the articulation of the AZT paradigm. During the initial years of the epidemic, the media consistently stressed that AIDS was not a manageable, let alone a curable, disease. "AIDS Cure May Prove Impossible," claimed the headline of a report in the *Cincinnati Enquirer* on October 23, 1985. Conjuring the image of the HIV's "clever mechanisms for infiltrating the body and jamming the disease-fighting immune system," the report, like many others at the time, emphasized the impossibility of a cure. Yet, at the same time, it quoted Dr. Luc Montagnier's view that "the best anyone could hope for was a combination of drugs to prolong the lives of patients." Suddenly, "prolonging lives" and "curing" were conceptually separated.

In general, the media's construction of AZT has uniformly affirmed this separatist view. When AZT was released, typical news headlines included: "U.S. Approves Drug to Prolong Lives of AIDS Patients, Cure Still Not Achieved" (*New York Times*, March 21, 1987); "AIDS Drugs Offer Hope but Cure Remains Distant" (*New York Times*, March 17, 1987); "AZT Offers Hope, but Not a Cure" (*Tampa Tribune-Times*, March 27, 1988).

Are curing and prolonging lives incompatible concepts? Their separation arises from the profound ideological difference between the model of a definitive eradication of diseases and the model of health management. From this difference emerges an important conceptual division with powerful implications for thinking about treatment: the idea of eradication purports to mark definitive differences between health and disease, while the idea of health management seeks to contain and regulate a reasonable level of health. But when measured against death, prolonging lives is no less significant than finding a cure. And when measured against the primary, localized need for health management and against the concrete obstacles to completely eradicating HIV, prolonging lives is obviously more desirable than lingering for a magical cure. As historian Allan Brandt has questioned: if the modern medical paradigm—the magic-bullet logic—has not worked to eradicate the crisis of venereal diseases that preceded AIDS, why would one believe that it would work for this particular infectious disease? (1987, p. 203).

One of the primary conflicts between AIDS scientists and AIDS activists emanates from this distinction between curing and prolonging lives. AIDS activists have long demanded a nonseparatist approach to AIDS care that would combine scientific drug and vaccine research with medical attention to clinical experiences, including attention to treatment for secondary infections. ACT UP's injunction—"Drug trials are health care too"—articulates the need for this bifocal approach to AIDS treatment. It argues that scientific intervention must continue and must be valued, provided that it merges research with health care, curing with prolonging lives (ACT UP, 1988, 1990a). The movement to use alternative, unorthodox treatments is also in part a response to this mystified separation (see chapter 2).

This argument characterized the AZT story until around 1989, foreshadowing a debate that emerged at that time in full force. As a result of challenges posed by scientists who were working on treatment for chronic diseases such as cancer, mental disease, diabetes, and heart disease, AZT found itself in a social terrain characterized by an increasing weakening of the traditional faith toward a single "technical fix" theory (see Eisenberg, 1986; Fox, 1992; Todd, 1990). The politics of AIDS underwent an important change in 1989, due to the shift of attention by health-care professionals and the public, who began to consider HIV infection as a chronic disease (Fox, 1992). This shift transferred the language of "chronic AIDS diseases" from the grass-roots level to the mainstream. Specifically, in the summer of 1989 the approval of aerosolized pentamidine for treating pneumocystic carinii pneumonia (PCP) and the finding that early use of AZT postponed the onset of symptoms in certain patients ushered in the new chronic disease paradigm. These events, however, did not dismantle antiviral AIDS research (nor should they have). AZT and AZT-like research continued. Medical historian Daniel Fox comments:

> By the late summer of 1989 . . . AIDS had been normalized, but in a somewhat different way than advocates for according it higher priority had expected. The response to the disease was now part of the normal fragmentation and frustration created by our health policy and disproportionately shared by the forty to fifty million Americans who lacked minimal health insurance coverage and by the health and policy professionals who addressed their needs. (1992, p. 128)

It seems that what occurred in the normalization of AIDS was its folding, as a chronic disease, into a chronic health-care crisis, a symbolic alteration of the popular meaning of the AIDS crisis without a concomitant alteration of the scientific paradigm in AIDS treatment research. What occurred was a move from the attention on research activities aimed at treating HIV infection to the focus on public-health activities associated with the AIDS crisis. The difference lies in a shift of the discursive terrain: the specific problem of AIDS treatment became the general discussion of health care.[6] In this way, the chronic disease model did not replace the magic-bullet model; they began to coexist. Did this coexistence—this bifocal emphasis urged by AIDS activists for some time—broaden the treatment possibilities? Yes and no.

The continuation of AZT research (i.e., the perpetuation of the AZT paradigm of treatment research) and the revitalized debate about health-care issues between 1989 and the present illustrate this coexistence. The approval in the summer of 1989 of early use of AZT made probable the continuation of AZT research in the coexisting paradigms. On the one hand, the idea that AZT could postpone the onset of symptoms marked HIV disease as a chronic health-care issue (and therefore justified its normalization). It even raised interest in developing prophylactic medicine. On the other hand, it kept intact the dominant research agenda, which embraced the AZT/antiviral/magic-bullet paradigm. Coincidentally, the discovery of HIV's mutating ability around the same period constituted a happy consistency with this discursive fold. HIV remained the key player—in fact the only player—in the world of AIDS treatment science; the only difference was that the play had been lengthened and the main character changed costumes more often now. Within this context, the medical vision for treatment was open and closed at the same time. In mainstream, federally funded AIDS treatment research, the clinical drug trial protocols remained firmly centered on the AZT paradigm, while the development of prophylactic and immune-boosting medicine received increased but peripheral attention (see Arno and Feiden, 1992).

Once again, we must realize the centrality of the AZT story and examine the perpetual confusion over its value under the symbolic and material conditions I have attempted to sketch here. Two things are certain so far. First, the confusion, controversies, and debates about AZT were not only about its material efficacy, as if how useful the drug is can be determined outside the framework that validates a certain thought pattern regarding therapeutic intervention, a certain social line of debate regarding the priorities of science, or a certain market formation. Second, in a more specific sense, AZT is caught in the middle of the "fold" between the magic-bullet model and the chronic disease model. It is little wonder that AZT is glorified and demonized simultaneously: a glorified demon.

## A Chronological and Media History of AZT

What are the important signposts and landmarks in the scientific creation of AZT? What are the conflicting forces prefigured and now contained in this creation? What forces stand to benefit from it? What role has the media played in its construction? What overall social debates and anxieties has it produced? These are some of the questions that articulate AZT as a historical force. They are linked, inevitably, to the important question regarding many AIDS patients' medical treatment decisions. How are AIDS patients to confront the conflicting accounts of AZT?

How would they make the necessary medical decisions regarding AZT, until recently the only approved antiviral drug around? My contention is that the discourse of impasse centered on the AZT story—which persists today—is a consequence of the conjunctural shifts in the cultural perception of technomedicine's authority, specifically the authority of the bio- medical paradigm conceived and practiced in AIDS treatment research and the authority of the marketplace model in the U.S. pharmaceutical industry. The confusion about AZT's actual usefulness or efficacy cannot be explained by the drug's chemical value alone.

To add a slightly different inflection to Pasteur's famous statement "The bacterium is nothing—the terrain everything," I have been suggest- ing a similar theoretical treatment of AZT. We need an archaeology of the AZT terrain in order to decipher its historical formations, the space of medical practices it constitutes and by which it is constituted, and the power it restores. To sketch this archaeology, I have combined the "offi- cial history" of AZT provided by Burroughs Wellcome, the pharmaceuti- cal company that researched and marketed the drug, and a "popular his- tory" rising from the media and activist protests. This chronology covers the period from the drug's first discovery until some of its latest develop- ment at the time of this writing, and includes the key events, players, and moments in the AZT terrain.

| | |
|---|---|
| 1964 | AZT was synthesized by Burroughs Wellcome (BW) as a potential cancer treatment but kept on the shelf soon after it was determined to be too toxic for human use. The researcher, Dr. Jerome Horwitz, along with AZT, was to be resummoned twenty years later on the ABC evening news as "Person of the Week" (March 27, 1987). |
| 1981 | BW prepared AZT for study as a potential human antibacterial agent. |
| March 1983 | CBS ran the first story on network television news explaining the problems in finding a cure for AIDS. The story focused on a possible breakthrough in pri- mate research. |
| June 1984 | BW began an AIDS research program to search for chemical compounds that might be effective against |

HIV. Five months later, AZT was identified as potentially useful against HIV.

Spring 1985     In vitro activity of AZT against HIV was confirmed by laboratories at Duke University, the Food and Drug Administration (FDA), and the National Cancer Institute (NCI). BW began toxicologic and pharmacologic testing of AZT.

June 1985     FDA permitted BW to begin clinical trials of AZT in humans.

July 1985     AZT was designated an orphan drug for the treatment of AIDS.

November 1985     CBS ran the first report on AZT on network television news. It contained an interview with Dr. Sam Broder of NCI and a testimony by patient John Solomon.

December 1985     BW began a collaborative Phase 1 study with NCI, Duke University, University of Miami, and University of California, Los Angeles, involving 40 patients.

February 1986     BW began a Phase 2 study at twelve academic centers, involving 281 patients. Trials were usually randomized, double-blinded, and placebo controlled.[7]

March 1986     ABC interviewed John Solomon and focused on research in Paris concerning restoring the body's immune system.

September 1986     The Phase 2 study was halted when an interim analysis showed a significantly lower mortality rate in patients who were receiving AZT compared to those randomized to receive a placebo. This incident was connected with the controversy already under way over the ethics of placebo trials.

September 1986     A cluster of coverage on AZT appeared on all three network news, citing Dr. David Barry from BW and Dr. Robert Windom, assistant secretary of health, who cautioned against overoptimism; Dr. Mathilde

Krim (American Foundation for AIDS Research, or AmFAR) and Dr. Paul Volberding (San Francisco General Hospital), who were hopeful and who praised the development; and three patients—John Solomon, Jon Stewart, and Bill Mason—who described their post-AZT conditions.

October 1986    FDA, the National Institutes of Health (NIH), and BW established a Treatment IND program as a means to provide wider access to AZT prior to FDA clearance.

March 1987    The FDA approved RETROVIR brand zidovudine (AZT) as a treatment for advanced AIDS-related complex and AIDS. The cost to patients would be $8,000 to $10,000 a year. Phase 3 was waived. The drug was two years in the approval process, which Frank Young of the FDA called the "irreducible minimum."

March 1987    *Science* magazine published Gina Kolata's "Imminent Marketing of AZT Raises Problems," which focused on the toxicity of the drug and why a majority of patients might not benefit from it. Already, doubts had been cast by the notorious *New York Times* reporter.

March 1987    The article "The FDA's Callous Response to AIDS," by Larry Kramer, founder of ACT UP (AIDS Coalition to Unleash Power) and cofounder of Gay Men's Health Crisis, appeared in the *New York Times*, March 23. Kramer charged that the FDA "constitutes the single most incomprehensible bottleneck in American bureaucratic history" and argued that existing drugs less toxic than AZT (e.g., ribavirin, AL 721, ddC) are not released as speedily as is AZT.

December 1987    Upon activists' protests, BW reduced the price of AZT by 20 percent to $8,000 per year for full-dosage users.

January 1988     Frank Young of the FDA announced its new drug
                 review process, citing the case of AZT as the evolu-
                 tionary prototype of an expedited drug release
                 process.

May 1988         Larry Kramer's "An Open Letter to Dr. Anthony
                 Fauci" of the National Institute of Allergy and Infec-
                 tious Diseases (NIAID) appeared in the *Village
                 Voice*; Kramer angrily charged Fauci with numerous
                 counts of incompetence.

July 1988        The *New York Times* printed Philip Boffey's "FDA
                 Is Pessimistic on Drugs to Fight AIDS," in which
                 Boffey reported that Frank Young of the FDA pre-
                 dicted that only one or two successful therapies to
                 treat AIDS would be found by 1991.

January 1989     The *New York Native*, a gay magazine, printed John
                 Lauritsen's "On the AZT Front," parts 1 and 2,
                 which claimed that "AZT is poison." The *Native*
                 subsequently printed a series of reports by Lauritsen,
                 building a case against the use of AZT.

March 1989       *Science* magazine published results of three teams of
                 researchers who detected strains of HIV that had
                 become resistant to AZT. ABC and CBS picked up
                 the story.

April 1989       On April 25, Power Tools, an affinity group of four
                 members of ACT UP, dressed as businessmen and
                 gained access to the Burroughs Wellcome offices at
                 Research Triangle, North Carolina. They then
                 protested the company's charging an exorbitant
                 price for AZT and demanded that it be lowered by
                 at least 25 percent, sealing themselves inside an
                 office by bolting steel plates to the door frame and
                 then informing the media of the event.

June 1989        In the Fifth International Conference on AIDS, held
                 in Montreal, over 370 sessions were devoted to the
                 discussion of AZT and of potential combination

therapies using AZT and other analogues (e.g., Acyclovir, ddI, ddC).

August 1989     Controlled clinical trials indicated that certain HIV-infected early symptomatic and asymptomatic persons could benefit from AZT with fewer or less-severe side effects. This news quickly became a major rallying point for early HIV antibody testing urged by both mainstream medicine and some community AIDS groups (see, for example, Smith, 1989).

September 1989     On September 14, Power Tools once again staged a protest, this time at the New York Stock Exchange. Seven men dressed as bond traders entered the site smoothly and went to the VIP balcony, from which they dropped a huge banner that said SELL WELCOME. They were subsequently joined by other ACT UP protesters outside the building, and the media were also notified of the event. On the same day, ACT UP San Francisco and ACT UP London held demonstrations protesting BW's pricing policy.

September 1989     On September 18, BW reduced the price of AZT by another 20 percent to $6,400 per year for full-dosage users.

October 1989     BW established a Pediatric Treatment IND program, providing wider access to AZT for medically eligible children prior to FDA clearance.

November 1989     *Spin* magazine printed Celia Farber's "Sins of Omission"; she outlined the core arguments against the approval of AZT, including the unscientific practices in the initial trials, the host of side effects of the drug, and the insufficient documentation of the drug's efficacy at the time of its release.

November 1989     *PWA Coalition Newsline*, a grass-roots newsletter primarily for gays and people of color with HIV/AIDS, published Rob Schick's "The Crazy Case against AZT." Schick challenged that the claim that

"AZT is poison" was erroneous, citing twelve scientific studies conducted internationally that supported the usefulness of AZT. Ultimately, his argument rested on personal experience with the drug as the determiner of its usefulness.

March 1990    On March 2, the FDA formally approved a change in the labeling of AZT, expanding the indications for use of the drug to include all adults with HIV and an immune T-cell count of 500 or less. Such a recommendation had been urged by many activists and grass-roots physicians for some time.

May 1990    The FDA approved expanded use of AZT to children who had HIV-related symptoms or significant suppression of their immune systems as a result of HIV.

November 1990    *Fortune* magazine published "The Inside Story of the AIDS Drug" after an interview with officials from BW. The article portrayed BW as the victim of harassment by Congress and AIDS activist groups.

January 1991    ABC reported that the U.S. government and two Canadian pharmaceutical companies had filed a lawsuit challenging Burroughs Wellcome's exclusive monopoly of the patenting of AZT. The government hoped that by listing itself as a coinventor of AZT, it could demand a share of profits. The Canadian companies sought patent ownership of AZT so as to distribute the drug at about one-third of BW's price and to spew competition. Two months later, a coalition of AIDS patients called Public Citizen also filed a lawsuit in federal court challenging BW's patent. Their aim was to bring down the price of the drug. ABC featured a two-part report of the lawsuit on January 2 and 3.

February 1991    Data released from a U.S. Veterans Administration (VA) cooperative study suggested that early treatment with AZT for persons with T-helper counts of

200 to 500 might not be helpful to blacks and Latinos, and might even be harmful. Racial difference in reaction to AZT, however, was not part of the original design of the trial. Scientists reviewing the VA study found the data "fragile" and suggested that such results might well be attributed to unlucky chance. Three months later, only CBS news among the three networks had picked up the story.

March 1991

On March 7, the Florida Department of Law Enforcement seized a supply of AZT and other medicines in a raid on the office of Trans-Aid, a community organization that gave away to patients who could not afford them AZT and other expensive medications left by someone who had died or by someone who had to discontinue use of AZT because of intolerance. Perhaps coincidentally, the raid took place during the AIDS hysteria in Florida springing from the Kimberly Bergalis story. Bergalis was the first person believed to be infected by a dentist, and this was considered to be an extremely rare mode of transmission. Her case sparked a feverish debate over whether medical personnel should be tested for the virus and whether their test results should be public information.

June 1991

*Nature* published "'Too Little, Too Late' for AZT," which assessed the recent flurry of legal challenges to BW's exclusive patent for AZT and suggested that none of the challenges appeared likely to change the pricing picture for AZT in the near future. Industry competition, it was reported, would be the factor that eventually cut the cost.

December 1991

The press reported a study that purported to show that the combination of AZT with an antiherpes drug, Acyclovir, resulted in a 50 percent reduction in the death rate of PWAs. The hype, as it turned out, was based on some misreporting, although it caused a $2 billion surge in the value of BW stock. The study had not been a combination trial at all, and the value of Acyclovir as an element in AIDS therapy remained uncertain.

February 1992    On February 13, the *New England Journal of Medicine* confirmed findings of the VA's Round 2 study of AZT (see February 1991 for results of the Round 1 study) that, although early treatment of AZT could slow the progression of AIDS, it did not prolong life. Researchers speculated that patients who took the drug early might develop resistance to it sooner than those who did not use early treatment.

February 1992    Harvard School of Medicine graduate student Yung-Kang Chow developed an idea for a new treatment by combining AZT with two other drugs. In vitro experiments indicated that this three-drug treatment seemed to damage HIV "beyond repair." The idea of combination therapy, which had been developing in recent years, crystallized in this new finding and might in turn have crystallized the chronic disease model in AIDS treatment.

April 1993    Yet another study argued that early treatment of AZT might not be of significant benefit to asymptomatic HIV-infected individuals. *The Lancet* reported an Anglo-French study, the Concorde trial, that used more end points in its determination of AZT's efficacy and lasted longer than all four similar U.S. trials combined.[8]

This chronology reveals a cluster of conflicting and unstable public images of AZT. The key themes include the spectacle of a "breakthrough" constructed around tales of pioneer innovation (such as that of Jerome Horwitz) and tales of endurance and leadership (such as Sam Broder's); the benefit of a strict observance of scientific standards through the clinical trial model and collaborative research; the politics of pricing and patent ownership; the ethics and politics of clinical trials; the perpetual pessimism with regard to drug development; the cautionary reactions; the enraged reactions (such as Larry Kramer's); the scandal of "poison"; the politics of research priority; and the rise and betrayal of hopes. Some of these themes are specific to the drug's history and clinical effects, but many arise from the diverse social, historical, political, and philosophical conflicts regarding technomedical practices in general, and AIDS treatment development in particular.

The ongoing quarrels within the scientific community, within activist groups, and between individual physicians and patients remain the central feature of the AZT story. Because so much is at stake—including scientific prestige, economic gain, and people's survival—the "success" story of AZT has been studded with disputes that still have not been fully resolved. Burroughs Wellcome's official history of AZT, which is packaged and distributed during International AIDS Conferences, has nullified many important points of conflict, as is evident in the press release "The Age of Antivirals: A New Era in Medicine" (see Burroughs Wellcome, 1990).

In this narrative milieu we witness the media's fluctuating coverage of "AZT science" as being monumentally groundbreaking at one moment and woefully disappointing at the next. The media's treatments of the British "AZT plus Acyclovir" story in 1991 and of the VA's Round 2 study of AZT in 1992 typify this contradiction.

In covering the British study, the media claimed unprecedented success for the combination therapy. The *London Times*, for instance, claimed that the AZT plus Acyclovir therapy promised to make the disease "completely treatable," and that it was the "most important find of the last ten years" (quoted in Project Inform, 1992, p. 10). The media in fact mistook the original intent of the study as an AZT plus Acyclovir study; it really was only a study of Acyclovir's value in preventing CMV retinitis (an eye infection that strikes patients in advanced AIDS). Coincidentally, the patients were permitted to use or not use AZT at their discretion. The study explained that only in a retrospective analysis did researchers find a differential death rate between those who were given Acyclovir and used AZT on the side and those who were given a placebo and used no AZT. With such preliminary and accidental findings, the media's erroneous claim of a causal relationship between using the two drugs and improved survival once again confirms its tendency to gravitate toward dramatic and simplified news. It also demonstrates the powerful seduction of the magic-bullet paradigm of medical treatment still subscribed by the popular imagination.

In the coverage of the VA study, the media misreported—in a gross simplification—that AZT had no value for early intervention against

HIV disease, when in fact the study merely demonstrated that early or late use of AZT yielded no significant difference in life expectancy (see Project Inform, 1992, p. 9). Such results are a far cry from saying that AZT is ineffective. Project Inform, a grass-roots AIDS organization based in San Francisco, commented that "the media dropped the bomb and quickly went on to the next story, leaving behind a wake of very distressed people more confused than ever about therapy" (p. 9).

Commentaries about AZT in the gay press and in community newsletters tend to fall into two categories: those that reject AZT on the basis of technical, scientific, and social investigations (Macanni, 1990; I. Young, 1988) and those that support AZT on the basis of individual clinical experiences (Project Inform). Sometimes this division is referred to as the "East Coast-West Coast conflict" of interpretation. As part of the cultural narratives of AZT, these views may serve to destabilize any unified truth claims about the drug. But they may also intensify the confusion that cripples people's medical decisions. The gay press has contributed to the anxiety over AZT.

For instance, John Lauritsen's writings between 1987 and 1989, collected in *Poison by Prescription: The AZT Story* and printed by the *New York Native*, represent a discourse of AZT resistance. Lauritsen's argument that AZT is poison reflects the overall position of the *Native*.[9] In a roundtable discussion on AZT organized by the *Native* in 1989, all the participants shared the view that "the government's administration of AZT to people with AIDS is genocide" ("Native Roundtable," 1989, p. 17). Presented as a forum for exploring the AZT controversy, that discussion did very little exploring but a great deal of consensus building.[10] One participant, Charles Ortleb, the publisher of *Native*, had this to say:

> The whole thing is punitive; AZT is in fact a punishment for being HIV positive basically. I think there's a general terror of just quickly ending the epidemic, there's a right-wing terror that people will go back to their wicked ways. The epidemic is seen by behavioral scientists as having a carrot and a stick: the carrot is you don't die if you don't get infected, the stick is you get poisoned with AZT if you do get infected. (p. 17)

This comment, of course, cannot attend to the need of many infected individuals actively struggling with treatment options. Other roundtable participants accused the AIDS treatment activism movement of assisting in the approval of AZT. For instance, Neenyah Ostrom, the managing editor of the *Native*, stated, "People keep saying, 'I'm not a scientist, I can't question HIV or Robert Gallo's work.' But those very same people feel capable of saying, 'Give me this drug, make this drug available now.' They don't say I'm not a scientist, I can't decide whether this drug is good for me or not" (p. 19). Such comments of course neglect to acknowledge that the fight for treatment requires activists and people with AIDS to wrestle with and intervene in all possible ways and that "making treatment decisions" is precisely that complex area that must not be left to scientists alone. Most ironically, the real contradiction in the discussion rests, on the one hand, in its overall distrust of the official scientific evidence that supports the effectiveness of AZT and, on the other hand, in its blatant reification of scientific rationality as the legitimate form of intervention.

To challenge the effectiveness of AZT requires an understanding of the deeply contested terrain where people are already situated, and where their individual priorities must be sorted out. Individual decisions are what Lauritsen's reports have disregarded. His discourse presents four main problems. First, he frequently draws on a conspiracy theory and problematic analogies. For example, he often compares AZT research to McCarthyism and Nazism. This is most apparent in his report of the State of the Art Conference on AZT Therapy for Early HIV Infection sponsored by the National Institute of Allergy and Infectious Diseases (see Lauritsen, 1990). Second, he questions the scientific validity of the AZT studies with little or no challenge to the fundamental scientific apparatus that drives them. For instance, although the bias of the controlled placebo method has been widely criticized, Lauritsen pays no attention to it. Third, he suggests that patients' own experiences of AZT do not substantiate the effectiveness of the drug (Lauritsen, 1989c). Finally, he offers no alternative suggestion to AZT. Lauritsen's voice was for a while echoed in the grass-roots movement, though his was certainly not the only interpretation offered by the gay community [see, for example, Schick (1989b) for an argument for AZT]. Alternative sources of commentaries were therefore not immune from the overall discourse and its deep-rooted controversies.

From the chronology of AZT, it is clear that Burroughs Wellcome has also been at the center of controversies. The debate over its pricing policy for AZT, for instance, would normally be determined by the sovereignty of the marketplace and the clout of the medical profession. Yet the very people most affected by the limited distribution of AZT (a result of its exorbitant price) refused to allow their fate to be controlled by the universality of the market. The protests by Power Tools in April and September 1989 not only put into question the universality of the market but lay bare a significant political perspective ignored by Burroughs Wellcome (and at times by the entire medical enterprise): that a crisis situation exists, and therefore the practices of medicine cannot be carried out in a business-as-usual manner. Some of the agonizing realities of the AZT story that have compounded the tensions of a whole social crisis about whose rules, whose sovereignty, we are to live by include Burroughs Wellcome's adamant refusal to open its books to justify its pricing policy, the seventeen-year exclusive right granted by the U.S. Patent Office to the company to manufacture AZT and control its price, and the murderous effect that the unreasonable price of AZT has had on the poor, on people of color, and on people in many developing countries.

A subtext of this conflict is the social struggle over libertarian control of the economics and dissemination of technology, and hence the control of biomedical knowledge. The ongoing challenge to Burroughs Wellcome's exclusive patent control of the AZT market again demonstrates this point. True, such challenges reinscribe the typical drama within the medical world over questions of prestige, honor, and profit, but this is not the only force at work. The peculiar coalition involving the government, private pharmaceutical companies, and active citizen groups comprised of AIDS patients and their advocates, all attempting to dismantle Burroughs Wellcome's AZT monopoly, suggests diminished social tolerance of the paradigm of the "free market" systematically reinstalled by the deregulation policies of the Reagan years. More specifically, it reveals the way AIDS activists, consumers, and advocate groups "get smart" in forming strategic alliances with different factions of the medical enterprise and mainstream health policy bodies in order to forge change in the pricing policy of AZT and thus critically challenge the mode of distribution and availability of the drug.

Meanwhile, the press, which has consistently ignored the activist protests (Crimp and Rolston, 1990, p. 117), has tended to manage the conflict by portraying Burroughs Wellcome as the victim of harassment. An article in *Fortune* in November 1990 opens as follows:

> They expected to be heroes—or at least to be appreciated. In the race to find a drug to fight AIDS, researchers at Burroughs Wellcome ran the pharmaceutical equivalent of an under-two-minute mile. In 1987, just three years after scientists learned what caused AIDS, the company won government approval for AZT ... in a fraction of the usual time. ... But

like the honor student who always does his homework but gets pushed all
over the playground at recess, Burroughs found itself ill prepared for the
explosive emotions and roughhouse politics surrounding AIDS. . . . The
heat Burroughs Wellcome endured seems more appropriate to a two-bit
toxic waste hauler with a malodorous history than to one of the world's
oldest, most respected drug companies. (O'Reilly, 1990, p. 113)

There is no dispute that Burroughs Wellcome did its "homework," but
no one knew that it was going to be tagged with a staggering price. The
image of the bullied victim, ironically, announces Burroughs Wellcome's
ignorance regarding the rapidly growing antiauthoritarian sentiment at
the time of massive government apathy toward the plight of people with
AIDS. It cannot expect to dominate play without knowing the climate of
the playground.

Like a good business confidant, the *Fortune* article goes on to offer
friendly advice to the company. According to *Fortune*'s analysis, Burroughs Wellcome lacks a proper public relations image: "Burroughs suffered most from not having a 'face,' a highly visible figure who could
demonstrate that the company cared about the suffering and the financial
consequences of AIDS." Specifically, it hints that the company "never
hired any openly gay people to explain why the price of the drug was
high or how it was being tested" (p. 128). Thus, in *Fortune*'s estimation,
Burroughs Wellcome was not a politically correct company.

Like Burroughs, *Fortune* fails to acknowledge that the epidemic long
ago had reached crisis proportions and that the usual commercially
sound business sense is precisely the core of the problem. The protest by
Power Tools at the New York Stock Exchange, crystallized in its banner
hung over the balcony: "SELL WELLCOME," underscores the reality, with
mortal stakes, that as long as Burroughs Wellcome continues to be "in
business" (that is, protected by the unchallenged universality of the marketplace, specifically the offensive calculation of business sense to determine the fate of a great number of people), AZT will remain out of reach
of many people in need, and will thus further compound the inherent difficulties of getting treatment because of demographic differences, particularly class and gender differences.[11]

Based on these observations, the AZT chronology can be read as both
a diagnosis and an inquiry. It closes and opens the AZT terrain simultaneously. On the one hand, it reveals that consensus is far from achieved,
by any stretch of the imagination. Conflicts, tensions, and schisms are the
central features of the story. Especially between 1987 and 1990, there

was little agreement about AZT's effectiveness, the debates inevitably centering on how to interpret the historical and sociopolitical structure that created the drug.

On the other hand, during the same time, medical sciences proceeded with a massive investment in AZT research. The media colluded in an intense focus on AZT, overshadowing coverage of all other potential treatment research. The post-AZT mainstream biomedical research to develop AIDS treatment has largely continued to be business as usual, despite the obvious conflicts in the AZT story. Dressed up as a giant showcase, the AZT model has lent significant authority to the dominant structure of rationality dear to mainstream technomedicine, namely the magic-bullet antiviral treatment paradigm, whose authority remained intact despite the rising perception of AIDS as a chronic disease. One can argue that AZT represents a paradigmatic vision of a modern medical breakthrough, a vision of contradiction. This is an important argument of this book. The contradictory representations of AZT—and the resultant confusion—may illuminate a broader path of thinking that contains and may benefit from a folding together of contradictory beliefs, a path that resuscitates the power of technological, commercial, and regulatory medicine. The archaeology of the AZT terrain lays bare a major framework of discourse within which further scientific inquiries, media representations, public health practices, or any qualifications of such must take place.

## AZT in the Media (2): "Rediscovering" AZT

Public health practices inevitably enter into the discourse of AZT. Because the history of the drug is so entwined within a complex cultural process, AZT has the power to influence public health considerations. This requires a strategic maneuvering of discourse, however, and it is instructive to briefly consider another media text that seems to make probable such a maneuvering.

In August 1989, the Department of Health and Human Services announced that early treatment with AZT for asymptomatic HIV-carriers could delay the onset of symptoms, and that the federal government would help the states pay for early AZT treatment under both Medicare and Medicaid. Public discussions immediately focused on the need for more voluntary HIV antibody testing to determine if an early AZT treatment should be taken. The media picked up the story and generated a range of questions, emphases, and inferences around the relationship between AZT treatment and testing. The character of the whole terrain of the AZT discourse suddenly changed. A compelling reason for HIV status testing, in the name of "medical need," reappeared. Filtered through social and media commentaries, the news inevitably rekindled the tension between new promise and new uncertainty. All of this comprises ABC's *Nightline* program "AZT and AIDS," broadcast on August 17, 1989.

I want to suggest that the *Nightline* broadcast was in no way a response to the medical breakthrough itself (if this is at all possible). Rather, it commanded a field of arguments that, through the new under-standing of AZT's value, supports a wide disclosure of people's HIV sta-tus information. This, I argue, constitutes a politics of controlled outing, warranted in economic and medical terms.

A structured lead-in report and a participant discussion that appears to be unstructured constitute the usual format of "Nightline." The first segment commonly assembles and frames the questions to be discussed in the second segment. Unlike that of regular news programs, this format serves to exercise a kind of liberalism that combines "objective report-ing" with subjective discussion. Cool descriptions mingle with hot debates, usually mediated by a knowledgeable and aggressive anchor. That the program is broadcast live gives the discussion segment an impression of raw freshness. The anchor's preconceived set of questions is offered as a mechanism of demeanor control in case the discussion "gets out of hand."

In "AZT and AIDS," the lead-in report weaves together a montage of issues around AZT that structures the discussion segment that follows. The issues include AZT's high cost, the allegedly disproportionate spend-ing on AIDS compared to spending on other diseases, discrimination based on HIV status, the changing epidemiology of the disease, and AIDS prevention strategies.

The reactions of AIDS activists within the gay and lesbian communi-ties to the AZT breakthrough news and to AIDS in general serve as the pillar of the report. On the one hand, the report first notes that because of the new value of AZT, AIDS activists are forced to reconsider and in some ways to relinquish their long-held position against involuntary test-ing. Declaring that "[with AZT] AIDS no longer means certain, swift, wretched death," the reporter explains why people such as Richard Dunn of Gay Men's Health Crisis were actively encouraging voluntary HIV testing. On the other hand, it comments: "Finally, there is the question of where public health issues blend into politics, where the battle over gay rights may drown out issues of how to fight the illness." It continues by citing Dr. Elizabeth Whelan of the American Council on Science and Health:

> I'm encouraging the AIDS establishment, if you will, to do what they can to detach the so-called rights of homosexuals from the AIDS epidemic as a medical problem. And also to really tone down the rhetoric related to so-called gay rights and the advancing of a sexually liberated agenda. They are not necessary to prevent AIDS.

These two themes—the plea for an attitude change among gay activists toward testing and the need for a depoliticization of AIDS—shift the terrain of discussion from the question of AZT's value to a problematic of gay involvement in AIDS treatment issues. A "soft" approach, it seems to suggest, is now more appropriate. Attached now to a discourse about gay politics, AZT as subject matter quickly fades into the background.

The second segment of the program revisits many of the themes from the first segment. The participants include Anthony Fauci of the National Institute of Allergy and Infectious Diseases; Tom Stoddard, a law professor at New York University and head of the Lambda Legal Defense Fund; and Lorraine Day of the San Francisco General Hospital. I will focus on two important moments of the discussion.

First, Ted Koppel asks Fauci and Day a series of questions about the funding of AIDS treatment: Who is going to shoulder it? How do we justify to heart disease and cancer patients the "disproportionate expenditure of money on AIDS research"? Is it wise to allocate an additional six billion dollars to "the distribution of AZT not for a cure, but simply for the extension of life"? These questions seemed to imply that AZT could become a major financial burden for the government, and that perhaps an unwarranted amount of money had been spent in AIDS research as a whole.

Fauci, in his usual bureaucratic manner, gives no concrete response as to the source of funding for the new policy of AZT distribution; he merely suggests that the government is in the process of working out a plan to finance it. This prompts Stoddard to point out that Fauci's comment typifies the government's overall lack of planning:

> Nobody's planning. . . . City of New York needs, over the next four years, seven billion dollars—doesn't have it—to deal with people with AIDS. Doesn't have it. State of New York, no one's home. No one's listening.

Federal level, no one's been planning. It's been eight years. We knew at
some point there would be new treatments available and yet nobody's
home.

To this somewhat unexpected comment, Koppel turns to ask for Day's
response. Day takes up Stoddard's comment but redirects it, suggesting
that the lack of federal planning is revealed by too much emphasis on
treatment research and not enough on prevention. She argues, as she had
earlier on this subject, that widespread, mandatory testing is essential to
yield epidemiological information for planning:

> Well, we have to handle this epidemic in a medical way, not a political
> way. And the way we've handled other epidemics is to find out, for public
> health authorities, not for publication in the newspapers, who has the dis-
> ease. And then they'll be able to plan and do the appropriate things to get
> the disease under control. Without knowing who has the disease, they will
> never be able to get it under control.

As to what "appropriate things" to do with the epidemiological information, Day does not specify. Apparently, "efficient planning" means something radically different for Stoddard and Day. Whereas Stoddard's comment points out a politics of negligence, Day's comment demands the
depoliticization of AIDS to achieve effective scientific control. In this
exchange, a political economic lesson of treatment is delivered, constructing a context where treatment and testing enmesh.

The second important moment in the discussion begins with another
series of questions from Koppel: Is there a difference between "a willingness to take a voluntary test and making the results of those tests available for epidemiological studies"? "If indeed people are simply going for
voluntary tests to find out, 'Am I all right,' is that going to do anybody
any good in the larger sense?" Will there be a point when "people will be
willing to let [the testing result] information be used for the kinds of studies that are necessary"? The possible responses are clearly predictable
and indeed are contained in the questions. What must be noted is that in
these questions a sequential movement of an argument is apparent: from
differentiating between individual and societal benefits of testing to pro-
jecting a possible movement of general disclosure of testing results.
Underlying this argument is a taken-for-granted, utilitarian ideal that sit-
uates "the larger good" before the individual's. This second moment
therefore puts forth, unambiguously, the specific argument for publiciz-
ing testing results, an argument that has radically demedicalized the use

of AZT. Together, the two moments imply that the disclosure of identity—a medical outing of sorts—may become a prerequisite for justifying massive federal spending on AZT.

## Summary

The "scene" of AZT in the broader discourse about "curing" AIDS is an ambivalent one. Like a seduction, the AZT story contains an enchanting fear that, at least in the media texts and the technomedical contexts, might well be called traumatic. Indeed, as we shall see in the following chapters, it is not too much to claim that as the narratives of "curing AIDS" are scripted simultaneously in the spaces of hope/hopelessness, Fall/Redemption, science/antiscience, and so on, these contradictions may induce a powerful trauma that may resusitate the political imaginary of the technomedical control of the body.

At one level, the trauma of AZT is spawned from deep-seated contradictions and tensions within the network of institutions, individuals, and communities negotiating and fighting for treatment options. Perhaps this is the context for what Paula Treichler (1991) calls the struggle for a "radically democratic technoculture." At another level, the trauma of AZT is constituted by the discursive ambivalence about AIDS curability/ incurability that frames or encodes a persistent production and reproduction of anxiety in the popular imagination. We cannot dismiss the contradictory tendencies in the media's representations of AZT as mere journalistic incompetence and fecklessness. Why do these contradictions seem to have such consistent regularity (that is, the regular production of anxiety), as the AZT chronology illustrates? We must examine the broader field that seems to command the unstable constructions of AZT.

The treatment paradigm operating in technomedicine, which coexists in the promises of a magic-bullet model and a chronic disease model, has sanctified the sacred quest for anything that looks like AZT, as the FDA's approval of ddI and ddC in 1990 and 1991 indicates (but even that has been vigorously challenged). The remaining question, it seems, is how the tangled narratives of AZT—the deeply divided positions, the fragmentation of viewpoints, and all the confusion created—affect people's real medical decisions *within* a field of contradictions. Conflicts compel practical remedies; we deal with the complex realities of AZT by struggling to take sides. But taking sides requires an analysis of the terrain already structured by specific forces, relations, and positions. While cultural knowledges must be struggled over, medical decisions are concurrently

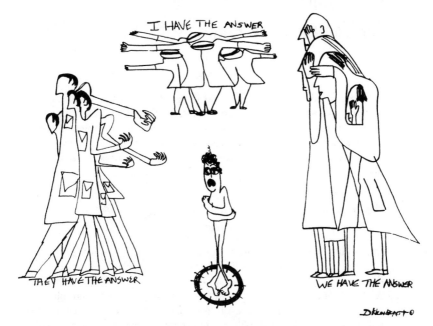

Figure 2.  Where is the answer? Reprinted with permission from *PWA Coalition Newsline*, December 1989, p. 34. The caption for the original publication read as follows: "Caring for one's health and choosing one's treatment is very stressful and confusing . . . what makes things even harder and more difficult is when people tell you they have the 'answer' and you haven't even asked the 'question'" (artwork and quotation by D. Kleinbeast).

and continuously made. How do we mediate between the two? How can we most effectively wrest control of contradictions and tensions that are in part culturally produced so that they might assist us, concretely, in making the necessary medical decisions? And, reciprocally, how do we carefully make those decisions with a concrete understanding of the (over)determinations of medical practices?

A cultural impasse—and the trauma it induces—is a condition that obstructs our ability to solve these problems effectively. It is the remarkably messy terrain that, while destabilizing all-encompassing narratives, may end up obstructing material decisions that have to be made. The real questions—Should one take AZT? When and in what clinical conditions should one start an AZT treatment or any other treatment?—remain firmly edged in the periphery of the doubtful mind, a condition of an (im)possible traumatic seduction.

# 2 Articulating the (Im)possible: The Contradictory Fantasies of "Curing" AIDS

> Nothing could be more meaningless than a virus. It has no point, no purpose, no plan; it is part of no scheme, carries no inherent significance. And yet nothing is harder for us to confront than the complete absence of meaning . . . for meaninglessness isn't just the opposite of meaning, it is the end of meaning and threatens the fragile structures by which we make sense of the world.
>
> Judith Williamson, "Every Virus Tells a Story"

> HIV/AIDS education must always be political.
>
> Cindy Patton, *Inventing AIDS*

> In our culture . . . the phobic narrative trajectory toward imagining a time *after the homosexual* is finally inseparable from that toward imagining a time *after the human* . . . . One of the many dangerous ways that AIDS discourse seems to ratify and amplify pre-inscribed homophobic mythologies is in its pseudo-evolutionary presentation of male homosexuality as a stage doomed to extinction (read, a phase the species is going through) on the enormous scale of whole populations.
>
> Eve Kosofsky Sedgwick, *Epistemology of the Closet*

*The AIDS Quarterly,* a television series created by PBS in 1989, opens with the following narration, backed by a solemn sound track reminiscent of the sound effects of a detective or horror film:

> The human immunodeficiency virus is not, in the strictest sense, a form of life. Until it is inside a host's body, it is no more alive than a rock or a stone. It is a protein-coded mass of genetic instructions 150 times smaller than the white blood cell it attacks. After penetrating, it multiplies until the cell bursts and dies. This continues for years. Cell by cell, the virus destroys its carrier's immune system. The person becomes ill from a series of infections that are progressively serious and rare and finally fatal. This is AIDS.

This narrative is accompanied by an image of the HIV, electronically colorized dark blue and green constantly shifting hues and intensities. A mediated spectacle is thus created, bound by the conventions of the representation of a mystical reality, projected as a new truth, and mobilized as a new frontier to be conquered. Since the onset of the AIDS epidemic, the HIV has become the center of an electrifying biomedical and cultural imagination, full of grave implications. Technoscience has made it possible to visualize and speak about this new truth. Yet, as the narrative indicates, it is, at best, an ambiguous truth: HIV is both lifeless and actively alive. It is a graspable, seeable, and somewhat innocent reality (as common as a rock or a stone) but simultaneously an unfamiliar object, a concept that exists only in the eyes of technology, a life-threatening entity beyond our control. Contradictory cultural constructs like this pervade the popular understanding of the discourse of AIDS treatment.

HIV is an especially potent cultural metaphor as much as it is a biological entity; the implications and consequences of each path of imaginings—let alone this duality—can be unpredictably varied and acute.[1] We cannot know in advance, for instance, the necessary effect of staging a clinical definition of HIV during a heated debate over the efficacy of a certain experimental drug, or in the context of a friend trying to help others to cope with the sudden news of their HIV seropositivity, or during a negotiation for safer sexual practices in the moment of intimacy. Nor can we always confidently assess the effects of revealing the weighty flow of cultural evocations surrounding HIV in varied social, cultural, political, or personal spaces. What seems important is the specific context, the specific trajectory within which the active imaginings of AIDS/HIV take a particularly strong foothold upon the knowledge projected in that context. One such context is the discourse about "curing" AIDS.

It would be misleading, however, to deny that meanings active in one domain of knowledge are not also active in another, or that they are not already reflexively active in a larger, more pervasive structure of meaning. In the discourse about "curing" AIDS, HIV (both its clinical and metaphoric realities) is central yet not entirely determining. The metaphoric evocations that have saturated around HIV are particularly abundant and potent in casting important and masterful definitions of the curability of AIDS. Yet such evocations are in turn overdetermined by the immense productiveness of the various constellation of fantasies surrounding the entire AIDS crisis, including, but not limited to, what I call the fantasy of menace and morbidity on the one hand, and the fantasy of control and containment on the other. These dominant fantasies have appeared to be potently systemic in its spread through all the veins of the mass media, medical publications, international conferences, classroom discussions, and so on.

Still, the contradictory images and narratives of HIV, such as the one created in *The AIDS Quarterly*, are central to the definition of the curability of AIDS, so that before one determines what to use to cure AIDS or how to cure AIDS, one must first negotiate, by analysis and intuition, the contradictory meanings of HIV. The stunning achievement of such contradictory meanings is the emergence of the conflicting, if not paradoxical, definitions of the curability/incurability of the disease, which depend of course on contextual usages but more importantly on the hyperemotive ideological tour de force of the fantasy structures just mentioned. Put another way, the social constructedness of HIV [which Paula Treichler (1992) has so eloquently analyzed] gives rise to perceptions of a relative potency/impotency of the virus—a matter that is a point of bitter debate among scientists today. But such perceptions would find it excruciatingly difficult to establish widespread credibility if they had not been overdetermined by the two ruling structures of fantasies of AIDS in our culture.

The fantasy structure of morbidity proliferates paranoiac identification of menace and emotional moribundity, bound by a series of morbid narratives, including most visibly the constructions of HIV as monstrosity, the intensively visual depictions of the disfigurement and wasting of the body, the horrifying statistical projections and death counting, the fantasy of "gay genocide," and of course the trauma of AZT.

The fantasy structure of containment, while consistently admitting the difficulty of finding a cure, couples curing with controlling in a regime of maximized hyperrationality. It too is enacted within a discursive boundary that activates—or habitually resuscitates—a set of narratives, including most visibly the ongoing coverage of AIDS drug and vaccine development; the mobilization of "AIDS education" campaigns, often condensed to the highly ambivalent injunction "Knowledge = Cure"; and the institutionalization of a rhetoric of reform of the technomedical paradigm of drug research and regulations. Such narratives have occasionally found support, rather peculiarly, in the keen observation of Wall Street's performance around AIDS drug development, so that economic performance may also serve as a sociopsychological index for the relative success of AIDS control. In addition, there is an ongoing attempt to disqualify any alternative forms of treatment, the effect of which is to control a particular visionary paradigm of containment deemed essential to the "proper" development of AIDS treatment.

This regime of control/containment focuses on the strategic conviction that while rationality, control, the constriction of behavior, even the repression of desire will not directly constitute a cure, they can lengthen the time and reconstitute the spaces deemed respectably necessary for controlling the disease. Although I do not assume stability in any of these strands of narratives contained in the fantasies of morbidity and containment, I am convinced that they have profoundly circumscribed the entire question of "curing" AIDS—circumscribed, that is, the inauguration of the stable definitions of AIDS as both curable and incurable.

The discourse surrounding AZT has resulted in a kind of abandon, an agonizingly discouraging scene that at the same time has also been the portal through which a specific biomedical paradigm of treatment research is left largely intact and therefore regains authority. Again, it would be difficult for AZT to sustain such a central discursive position (defined neither as certain victory nor as absolute failure) were it not for the continuously massive cultivation of the fantasies of morbidity/containment. In this way, the overall bifurcated status of "curing AIDS" is characteristically organic.

## "AIDS Is Incurable": The Structure of Morbidity

If a masterful assertion and reassertion of the invincibility of AIDS can be made (and made with the passionate conviction we have witnessed in all these years of the epidemic), it has to be in large part incurred by the immensely figurative statement that "AIDS is invariably fatal"—figurative not because it is fictional but because, in a far more productive way, it abides by a looming fantasy structure of morbidity as it actively constructs the morbid scene. The statement "AIDS is invariably fatal" has been so central and so deeply permeated into every discourse, from the most austere professional scientific language to the news, that the site of its origin is no longer possible to locate.

The contention that "AIDS is invariably fatal," as opposed to "AIDS causes death" or just "AIDS is fatal," depends on the weighty inscriptions of the following truth claims, listed here in order of expanding intensity and complexity:

1. HIV *inevitably* causes AIDS.
2. Epidemiological information will *always* be unambiguously reflective of reality.

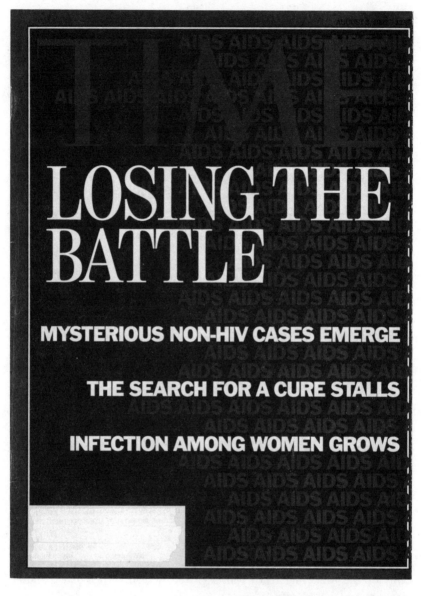

Figure 3. Representing despair. *Time*'s August 3, 1992, version of the "invincibility" of AIDS, represented in the cover design bearing the look of an AIDS invasion (always coded in red), an invasion even of the space between words.

3. Although HIV is thought to be vastly mutable, its infectivity will be *permanently* immutable; infection will be carried out in a permanent and progressive irreversibility.

4. Treatment will *inevitably* fail.

5. The manifestation of illness may not always be uniform, but death will be the *universal* result.

Each of the qualifying linguistic markers—always, permanently, inevitably, universal—must appear in these truth claims with spectacular force in order to anchor and naturalize the compelling clause "invariably fatal." At the same time, these qualifiers do not necessarily connote something already accomplished. In fact, the rigid inevitability they connote suggests a sense of something constantly in progress; they help to launch the more powerful assertion "It *will* happen" rather than "It *has* happened." Morbidity is always less of an achievement than a prospect.

The interconnecting (and competing) discourses of science, including virology, epidemiology, immunology, and clinical research, are the grounds for the inevitability suggested by the combination of "invariably" and "fatal." Two things give this combination its rhetorical force. The first is the creation of a linear momentum, a medical domino theory of sorts provided by the scientific definition of AIDS as consisting of several progressive and irreversible stages of deterioration, as evidenced by the elaboration of the theory of a temporally linear HIV life cycle and the epidemiological tracking of symptom development over time. The second is the creation of a specified destiny, namely the stage of "full-blown AIDS" ("full-blown" means "mature" and "large as life"), in which time has run out and life itself is replaced by deadly symptoms. Susan Sontag has written, "construing [AIDS] as divided into distinct stages was the necessary way of implementing the metaphor of 'full-blown' disease'" (1989, p. 29). The phrase "invariably fatal" therefore depends on the installation of a temporality of symptom development; it need not pronounce death itself in order to promise the prospect of death. The question of temporality in the discourse of curing AIDS is examined in detail in chapter 3.

To the degree that "AIDS is invariably fatal" means that "AIDS *will be* fatal," the tragedy becomes both more and less catastrophic, because fatality, in this statement, is being constructed to be at once a prominent and an imminent calamity. In speaking about the apocalyptic vision surrounding AIDS in general, Sontag has made a similar observation:

With the inflation of apocalyptic rhetoric has come the increasing unreal-
ity of the apocalypse. . . . A permanent modern scenario: apocalypse
looms . . . and it doesn't occur. . . . There is what is happening now. And
there is what it portends: the imminent, but not yet actual, and not really
graspable, disaster. Two kinds of disaster, actually. And a gap between
them, in which the imagination flounders. (1989, pp. 87–90)

Morbidity is an event that is happening and not happening. This gruesome reality of catastrophe/noncatastrophe (sudden tragedy/expected
tragedy) made probable by temporalizing the disease has therefore compounded its disease-ing. Sontag, after identifying the discursive ambiguity carried in the fatalistic view, nonetheless continues to use a language of
doom: "Now the generic rebuke to life and to hope is AIDS" (p. 24);
AIDS is "an unprecedented menace" (p. 85); it has inspired "the fantasies
of doom" (p. 87); AIDS is "extremely recalcitrant to treatment" (p. 16).
Ultimately, the yoking of AIDS, the permanent inevitability of disease,
and death fabricates a definition of its incurability and positions us in a
state of diseased reality.

AIDS = Death has been the basis of a constant proliferation of narratives and images of fatalism, brutal disfiguration of bodies, and grim projections that circulate in the orbit of the fantasy of morbidity. The construction of HIV as a monstrosity cannot in itself gain a permanently
secure footing upon the morbid imagination of the incurability of AIDS.
What seems to be at work is an endemic linkage of HIV with a series of
constructed social horrors, which generates an aura of maximum anxiety
around the AIDS menace.

### Spectacular HIV

Even though in recent years, as a result of increased understanding of the
disease, the plague model of interpretation has been shifted to the chronic disease model, suggesting that an extended survival period is now possible, the discourse about the horror of AIDS remains dangerously pervasive. New understanding has not shattered the intensive social discussion
of the HIV as the impossible obstacle in the scientific crusade against the
disease, the culprit of horror.

A virus is a biological entity as well as a socially produced text,
absorbed in the gaze of medical researchers, offered up by journalists as
the center of the mystery of AIDS. The visual image of HIV purports to

tell the "truth" of a complex reality; seeing literally becomes knowing (Grover, 1989; McGrath, 1990).

Milan Kundera has said: "Once we can name each part of our body, that body disturbs us less." But whether the discursive constructions of HIV—the "naming" of the AIDS body—disturb us less or not depends on how they are deployed and what audience they implicate. In fact, the emphasis on the widespread but "low-keyed" infectivity of HIV—the so-called silent infection—provokes fear in everyone; no one, it seems, is less disturbed. Overall, media and biomedical discourses construct HIV as the abhorrent figure, frequently invoking images of familiar characters in science fictions and detective stories:

- HIV is an insidious, indiscriminate killer.
- HIV is a time bomb, gradually wasting away its carrier's life.
- It has a brilliant genetic design that facilitates undetectable infection.
- Its genetic component replicates and mutates wildly.
- It is the invading battalion, turning the body into a war zone.
- It infects like a violent postmodern military attack.
- Its power lies in its ability to claim territories and remain there to reproduce its own kind.
- It knows how to hide itself in order to carry out its secret mission; it is the evasive Trojan horse.
- Eventually, it penetrates significant zones of the body.
- It evolves from a family of deadly viruses.
- Its origin is unmistakably foreign and alien; it either comes from subhuman species (monkeys) or from bizarre human sexual practices.[2]

Consider also this narrative by two leading biomedical researchers of AIDS:

> The picture is a daunting one. HIV is able to slip into cells and remain there for life. Its elaborate genetic regulation enables it to lie low, hidden from immune surveillance; to replicate slowly, possibly deranging the host cell's own genetic controls as it does so, or to initiate a burst of growth that kills the infected cell. (Haseltine and Wong-Staal, 1988, p. 62)

Detective story meets science fiction. In the popular lexicons of Star Wars, serial killing, perversion, and deception, the HIV has proved an ideally comprehensible subject. As the preceding listing suggests, the virus has become a coherent character, perfectly endowed with (malignant) intentions, purposes, schedules, targets, and even preferences (Williamson, 1989).

A journalist describes the HIV as "wandering through the world of life, looking for living cells to infect" (Schmeck, 1987). Similarly, a television special report called "AIDS Now" produced by Channel 4 in England features a detective taking on the case of a criminal suspect, the HIV. Coded in all the conventions of the detective story (dark, wet streets; dim lighting; mysterious music; and, of course, the detective in raincoat and hat), the investigation unfolds as the detective replays evidence on a video recording machine, looking for traces of the mysterious killer. Most of the prominent medical researchers, journalists, and social policy makers featured in the video express fear and pessimism about locating the killer or gaining information about its motives and its next attack. Sound familiar? More questions are asked than answers given, and the audience is left more disturbed than ever. The case is pending, more work is needed, and in the meantime the killer remains elusive. Throughout the program, the story of the HIV is named "The Case of a Promiscuous Parasite."

### "AIDS Body," "AIDS Statistics," and Morbidity

If the fantasy structure of morbidity revolves around temporalized notions of imminence, expectedness, permanent inevitability, and so on, then it also must depend on the constant marking and monitoring of charged sites of morbidity in the "AIDS body," marking, in a fairly literal sense, the body parts that are scientifically demonstrated to be the zones of infection/zones of horror and monitoring their imminent deterioration. The "AIDS body" therefore comes to stand for the literal and figurative object of the (in)curable in a journalistic and medical culture obsessed with morbidity.

The morbid constructions of the AIDS body as a horrific spectacle have been widely discussed (see, for example, Gilman, 1988; Grover, 1989; Landers, 1988; McGrath, 1990; Treichler, 1987). As Simon Watney has observed:

> The political unconscious of the visual register of AIDS commentary . . .
> assumes the form of a diptych. On one panel we are shown the HIV retro-
> virus (repeatedly misdescribed as the "AIDS virus") made to appear, by
> means of electron microscopy or reconstructive computer graphics, like a

huge technicolor asteroid. On the other panel we witness the "AIDS victim," usually hospitalized and physically debilitated, "withered, wrinkled, and loathsome of visage." . . . This is the *spectacle of AIDS*, constituted in a regime of massively overdetermined images. (1987b, p. 78; emphasis in the original)

This double sign—the "diptych"—weaves a spectacular drama consisting of the image of the miraculous, almost seductive, technological achievement of clinical medicine on the one hand, and the hyperemotional emblem of the emaciated body on the other, always focusing on the blistered and swollen face. The space between the layering of these two images is ideal for the staging of a curing narrative.

Susan Sontag, contemplating the cultural significance of the human face, suggests that Western culture's

> conviction of the separation of *face* and body . . . influences every aspect of manners, fashion, sexual appreciation, aesthetic sensibility—virtually all our notions of appropriateness. . . . Our very notion of the person, of dignity, depends on the separation of face from body, on the possibility that the face may be exempt, or exempt itself, from what is happening to the body. And however lethal, illnesses like heart attacks and influenza that do not damage or deform the face never arouse the deepest dread. (1989, pp. 39-40; emphasis in the original)

The privileging of the face thus holds up the superfluously prized aesthetics of human worth. As such, the deteriorated face not only mortifies the entire body, it also suggests a decomposition of character:

> What counts more than the amount of disfigurement is that it reflects underlying, ongoing changes, the dissolution of the person. . . . The marks on the face of a leper, a syphilitic, someone with AIDS are the signs of a progressive mutation, decomposition; something organic. (1989, p. 41)

Simon Watney has made a similar observation: "The outward and visible signs of infection [are] taken as evidence of their supposed inner and secret depravity" (1990, p. 173). The psychological fear caused by such a suggestive mutation originating from the face is what the conventional journalistic ritual of before/after photographs induce. Such a technique in photojournalism, though not unique to the representation of people with AIDS, has been especially crucial in mobilizing fear, particularly during the early years of the epidemic. Cases in point are the photographs that appeared after the revelation of Rock Hudson's illness in 1985, which focused on the physical transformation of Hudson's face and body, and the brutally manipulative television use of PWA Kenny Ramsaur's face before and after his illness in 1983 and of another PWA, Fabian Bridges, in 1985.[3]

In recent years, however, the "face of AIDS" has received a different treatment by the media. As political activism has grown and, to a smaller degree, as public outcry has expressed distaste for the dehumanizing staging of debilitated AIDS patients in the media, the emaciated face has gradually lost its powerful hold on the popular morbid imagination. Yet this trend has not by any means diminished attention to the face as a crucial trope for suffering, horror, and morbidity. The different treatment is in part a result of the normalization of AIDS alluded to in the last chapter, and from the same normalization process has sprung a more subtle but no less potent imaging of the "AIDS face" in the popular media.

Although use of the before/after convention in photojournalism has diminished, a modification of it can be found in *Time* magazine (August 3, 1992). A pair of photographs of the face of a hemophiliac child named Laurent (whose family name is, as usual, missing) before and after he was severely affected by HIV are not presented side by side, but separated. A photograph of his face, gaunt as a result of illness associated with AIDS, appears on the contents page, captioned "Laurent, pictured as a healthy child on page 31, died of AIDS earlier this year at age 11." As the reader is invited to turn anxiously to page 31, we are led, in a representational reversal (after/before), to a melancholic, even nostalgic, look at the pitiful. The grainy image of Laurent with his brother Stephane, who had also contracted HIV but was still alive, looks like a typical family portrait, advancing all the emotional melancholia promised by the convention of a family portrait. In the pair of images of Laurent, therefore, we are given, in a psychic reversal, a potent suggestion of fear: "Look, it used to be . . . " becomes a more powerful vantage point for soliciting the morbid imagination than "Look, it has become . . ." Of course, the portrait of Laurent and his brother Stephane also sets in motion the imminence of Stephane's expected fate, the promise of an implied prospect of an "after" image.

In recent years, we have encountered in the media largely a representational turn to the documentation of the "Faces of AIDS" in the media's self-reflexive attempt to counteract the dehumanizing effect of impersonal AIDS reporting. But the photographs of human faces usually appear in small, silent rectangles that fill the page and are, in such a layout, rarely accompanied by any meaningful information about the individuals represented in the bodiless, contextless images—what Simon Watney calls the "black-and-white testimonial space of the 'AIDS victim'" (1990, p. 183). Unlike the assemblage in the Names Project, they thus continue to transcend and mystify death. [4] Meanwhile, inventive images of silhouetted or digitalized faces of people with AIDS continue to be the ordinary practice of television news.

In 1992, in a highly controversial media advertising campaign, the face of AIDS, already immortalized in the photographic representations of the crisis as a whole, reappeared in the image of an AIDS patient on his deathbed in an immodest Benetton advertisement (fig. 4). Given the pervasiveness of the visual horror in the photographs of AIDS, few failed to recognize this as an image of a dying AIDS patient. By 1992, an image of a dying person with AIDS had become routine; no ethical answerability or prudence was thought necessary to accompany such an image. What is also routine, in the visual form in which the image is shaped, is that the dying person, David Kirby, is surrounded by family (belonging to the photographic tradition of a family portrait), and that this gathering takes place in a hospital or a hospice (the "natural" dignified sites of death). The collective cultural fantasy of family unity typified in such a portrait, even in a tragic moment, appears to be a point of cognitive articulation with the inventive message in Benetton's benign logo: "UNITED COLORS OF BENETTON."

As the advertisement has only appeared in photographic form (the Benetton campaign advertises only in magazines and on billboards), it marks the space of the dead redundantly. As Christian Metz has suggested, the photographic image—indeed, the photographic medium itself—abducts the object out of the world and transfixes it in the objectification of death, immortalizing the object in the memory of the dead *as being dead* (1990, p. 158). Nothing in the Benetton photograph is more culturally naturalized as the mark of death than the AIDS patient's gaunt, barren, emotionless face, a face that relinquishes consciousness and therefore relinquishes the space of the living. The common recognition that Kirby's face resembles that of Christ (the photographer's intent?) aligns, even by coincidence, this image with the space of extreme suffering fixed in Christ's face, which is, in Christian iconography, commonly recognized as the site of excruciating morbidity: at the moment of his abandonment, Christ suffers, and suffers only, in his face.[5] All the volatile suggestiveness of the image fortifies the morbidity so deeply articulated with AIDS.

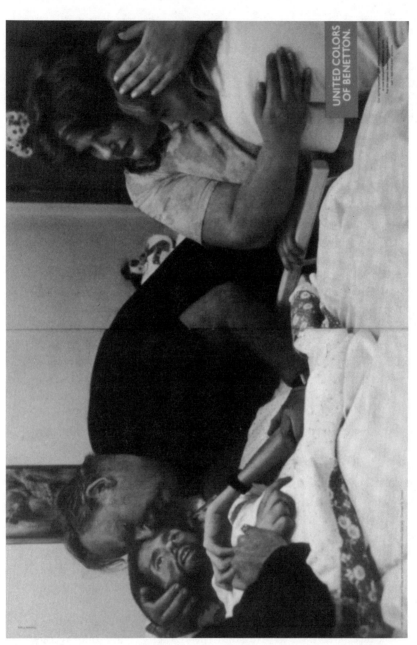

Figure 4. Selling Benetton. A Benetton advertisement features a dying AIDS patient with a Christ-like face. "Morbidity" centers on the representation of the face of a dying person. The face authorizes a subtle perception of how the outward and visible signs of suffering are taken as evidence of the individual's inner despair and capacity for atonement.

By locking the gaze of the reader onto Kirby's face while he in turn directs his own empty gaze toward somewhere and nowhere—he is already elsewhere—the image both seduces our attention and abandons it into a nonspace; it draws us toward a place where any meaning and no meaning can coexist. The image of Kirby, particularly his face, suggests that the space of the living *is being* evacuated, as opposed to *has been* evacuated, and therefore provides us with a prolonged glimpse at the abject trajectory of morbidity itself.

One may then say that the image's shock value lies in its normality, not the normality of the appearance of such an image in the pages of *Vogue, Cosmopolitan,* or *Details,* but the numbing shock of a glimpse of a morbid death associated with AIDS, the banal news in an unexpected space of a popular magazine. The main point of the public controversy surrounding Benetton's 1992 campaign echoed AIDS activists' long-held position: "No more pictures without context." No context is given to the image in the photo: no explanation of Kirby's story, no high-powered advertising pitch for Benetton's product (what product?). But the absence of context precisely constitutes the image's force. Conspicuously context-less but unavoidably overdetermined by the psychosocial context of the morbid, this shockingly normal (routine, naturalized, taken-for-granted) image exempts itself and is exempted from any explanation of its specific content. One thing is sure: the clothing company's immodest claim of a unified world (the point of such a unity remains highly ambiguous) represents its attempt to mimic the call for solidarity by political activist groups already mobilized around AIDS and other social crises. Concurring with, appropriating, or mimicking political activism, as Benetton's spokesperson has tacitly admitted, is rapidly becoming good corporate practice. As in the encompassing psychosocial contention that "AIDS is invariably fatal," in Benetton's advertisement the desire is to proliferate abject emotions toward the dying dead.

A strikingly similar photograph of another PWA, Donald Prenata, in which a loved one leans over Prenata's deathbed and kisses his forehead, appeared in the *Hartford Courant* (September 30, 1990). Prenata's face, like the face of the AIDS patient in the Benetton advertisement, suggests excruciating pain. His blank look—the "already elsewhere" look—again evacuates itself from the realm of the human symbolized by the embrace of the surviving loved one. From these images of visionary despondence (even despair over meaning), we see the growing dejection that continues to shape the imaginative definition of the incurability of AIDS.

At a more routine but scarcely less grievous level, the vision of incurability is continuously expressed in quantitative terms. Anyone who reads the news about AIDS is violently subjected to a concrete sense of despondence through ubiquitous reminders of its death toll, as in this passage from a *Newsweek* article (June 25, 1990), "AIDS: The Next Ten Years":

> A sense of crisis is hard to sustain. It thrives on earthquakes and tornadoes, plane crashes and terrorist bombings. But forces that kill people one at a time have a way of fading into the psychic landscape. So, if you've stopped thinking of AIDS as an emergency, consider a few numbers."(Cowley et al., 1990, p. 20)

Although considering "a few numbers" is hardly sufficient to regain and sustain awareness of the crisis, the force of the authors' instruction rests in the definition of AIDS as embodying "forces that kill people one at a time." Like the other calamities (earthquakes, tornadoes, plane crashes, and terrorist bombings), AIDS kills. But in this construction, unlike them, AIDS death is thought to occur with an implicit regularity. Reminders of AIDS death in the news—indeed, a morbid fascination with death—almost always resist a suggestion of speculation because that would mean randomness. Rather, AIDS death is always considered to be wholly predictable. Particularly in the news, AIDS casualty is almost never treated as catastrophic, which would suggest suddenness and shock. Indeed, the basis for an institutional force galvanized to body counting—such as the publication of *The HIV/AIDS Surveillance Report* produced by the Centers for Disease Control—is that AIDS death *is* predictable. Statistical models, not the reality of people dying of AIDS, invent the notion of AIDS death through a series of transformations: from a qualitative into a quantitative reality, from possibilities into probability, from an aura of catastrophe into the specter of information.

The constant appearance of grim projections regarding the future status of the crisis always seems to have something to do with the confrontation with an eager expectation (a fundamental character of morbidity) and its potential for technological inventiveness. Because of the fascination with death, the grim statistics might finally be defined as the conjuncture of technology and morbidity. There can be no counting *of* death without a technocultural emphasis that counts *on* death.

Yet, by virtue of methodology and presentation, the technology in this instance almost always guarantees a failure of understanding. What is usually presented is a projection fixed in the future by way of a conception of the present condition. In other words, statistical projections would not be possible without the manipulation of the conjuncture between the present and the future. To attempt a glimpse into the future might force preventive action on the present. Yet any preventive action would have to be justified by its efficacy, which is measured only by projection (back) into the future. How the conjuncture between the present and the future is manipulated may invite disputes among statisticians, which perhaps explains why presentations of AIDS statistics always seem to contain first a projected figure ("The officials say . . .") and then a comparison ("But other experts say . . ."). The two figures may be so disparate as to cause at least confusion and, as the second figure is almost always a revision upward, often the sense of a forever-escalating menace. What remains constant in this murky numerical trajectory is the appearance of expected, even deserved, death. The eager delivery of grim statistical projections of AIDS casualties may have something to do with the equally eager habitual affirmation that something wrong, unnatural, or perverse has been committed by someone. The transmissibility of surveillance information, therefore, depends wholly on the transmission of sexual or drug use behavior in predefined "exposure categories" among "high-risk" groups. Numbers in this way have the power to create identities, even subjects.

### The Fantasy of "Gay Genocide"

Perhaps the most lethal and spontaneous part of the morbid imagination about AIDS is the recondite, pervasive, and almost transcendental regard of homosexuality (particularly male homosexuality) as the morbid center of (self-)destruction. The deep codes of fear and repugnance that saturate the cultural fantasy of the *danse macabre* surrounding AIDS show up in the continual rupture, for over twelve years now, of an arsenal of lethal representations—that AIDS is "invariably fatal," that HIV is permanently monstrous, that all people with AIDS are the clinical embodiment of grotesque disfigurement (of both body and character), that AIDS statistics authorize the de facto sign of inevitable massive deaths. This atmosphere seems vindictively eager to imagine a historical prospect of the eradication of "homosexual acts," whether carried out by homosexuals or not, and, by extension, the eradication of the figure of the homosexual. Present within the fantasy structure of morbidity is the idea of, even a yearning for, a "cure" that would restore history, itself ravaged by the AIDS crisis, through an order of eradication. Eve Sedgwick has cast a similar hint as she traces the historical treatment of sodomy:

> There is the inveterate topos of associating gay acts or persons with fatalities vastly broader than their own extent. . . . there is a peculiarly close, though never precisely defined, affinity between same-sex desire and some historical condition of moribundity, called "decadence," to which not individuals or minorities but whole civilizations are subject. Bloodletting on a scale more massive by orders of magnitude than any gay minority presence in the culture is the "cure," if cure there be, to the mortal illness of decadence. (1990, p. 128)

What we have witnessed since 1981 in media reporting and government treatment of AIDS is the emergence, however uneven, of a condition that has reversed Sedgwick's qualifier "though never precisely defined" to describe the lethal association of gayness and death. It is not too much to claim that the convergent injunctions of "AIDS is a gay disease" and "AIDS is invariably fatal" have been inaugurated, with spectacular sovereignty, as the amalgamized definition of AIDS in all veins of popular and official rhetorics.

Such an indomitable psychocultural collapse of a disease syndrome, a whole culture of people, and guaranteed fatality—what Jeff Nunokawa (1991) calls "the aura of doom that surrounds gay men" and what PWA Meurig Horton (1989) refers to as the "vampiric state of the undead"— is perhaps the major strengthening force for the belief in the HIV's destructiveness. This morbid delineation of gay identity has effectively limited the space for alternative imaginings of the power of the HIV. Hence, quite possibly, there is an emergence of a thickening vision of a "cure" for HIV infection that is being driven toward the fantasy of gay genocide.

This evolutionary thinking in the current wave of morbid/genocidal fantasy has also lent support to, and in turn is supported by, the presumably corruptive power of gay men living with HIV/AIDS. Douglas Crimp argues that the obsessive delineation of gay PWAs as nothing but degenerating bodies is the result of a phobic terror that imagines them as still sexually active and, by implication, still willfully contagious (1992, p. 130). In the homophobic imagination, the end of "gay promiscuity," or perhaps of gay sex altogether, is therefore symbolically coherent with the idea of the extinction of the homosexual. One way in which the media eagerly invite us to feel infuriated at the "misconduct" of gay PWAs, and as a result to feel justified in eliminating them from our midst, is the construction of PWAs as victimizers of "innocent bystanders." In 1987 alone, the *New York Times* carried stories of sixteen incidents in which PWAs, mostly gay or bisexual men, appeared as the subjects of crime stories. Typical narratives portray them as villains who willfully infect others around them by "savage" acts of biting, spitting, scratching, and, the most unimaginable of all, soliciting unprotected sex without revealing their HIV seropositivity.[6] In these stories, an association between pathology and criminality—in congruence with the historical construction of madness—is made over the social caricature of gay PWAs, which hastens the hatred of gay men. The appearance of the malicious statement "AIDS Kills Fags Dead" on T-shirts, in dorm windows, on bumper stickers, and in other public spaces is a stunning, succinct statement of hatred toward "AIDS-ed" male homosexuals; a parody of the insecticide slogan "Raid Kills Bugs Dead," it provokes the consummate desire for the eradication of all gay men, like the eradication of roaches.

Similarly, in the summer of 1989 the San Francisco gay press published an image from a piece of hate mail distributed in the streets that summer (fig. 5). As is typical for hate mail, the face of AIDS is the face of a gay man, even though the leaflet was presumed to be aimed at lesbian ministers in the city. In this horrific image there is no subtle, soft homophobia counseling acquiescence to the tragedy of AIDS, no calm suggestion of a gruesome (self-)destruction. We will fail to understand the magnitude of the fantasy of gay genocide if we think it occupies only the minds of ruthless extremist groups, tough hoodlums, or deplorable figures such as Jesse Helms and Pat Buchanan. Subtle or not, calm or not, the fantasy, as exemplified in figure 5, swells to the clouds the delirious, and ultimately mad, contemplation of a human culture *after homosexuality*.

Lee Edelman's provocative statement that "there is no available discourse on AIDS that is not itself diseased" (1989, p. 316) should remind us of the variegated, but convergent, modalities and effects of all discursive work contaminated by the lethal fantasy of morbidity. An utterly homophobic culture that plots the amalgamation of gay sex, AIDS, and death must inter homosexuality in its entirety and dissociate it from the imagination of curing. If gay death is taken to be the basic, even banalized, tragedy in the historical crisis of AIDS, it is also inclined to be viewed as the basic necessity for "curing" a disintegrating historical order. If the homophobic culture widely regards treatment activism as

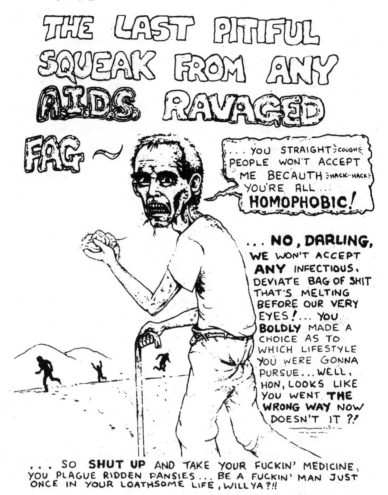

Figure 5. Hate mail. A homophobic leaflet thrown from a passing truck to a San Francisco street protest against the harassment and assault experienced by a lesbian minister in the summer of 1989. Reprinted from the *Bay Area Reporter* editorial page, August 3, 1989.

the gay movement's new agenda, then it also considers it axiomatic that a proper way to develop treatment for AIDS must contain a limitation of the effects of treatment activism (see chapter 4). In short, if homosexuality is the subject of the morbidity of AIDS, coded as imminent massive self-destruction, if not extinction, then nonhomosexuality becomes the object of curing. Within these relational discursive turns, we may begin to witness another powerfully active fantasy regarding the various imaginings of how AIDS can be "cured." This fantasy of control/containment can be viewed simultaneously as parallel to, and an effect of, the fantasy of morbidity.

## Science Fictions: The Fantasy of Control/Containment

Side by side with the overall construction of the impossibility of AIDS is a fantasy structure that proclaims the immense curative power of medical science to fight AIDS through a paradigm of hyperrationality. Through the years, the press has reported the steady supply of experimental drugs and new inventions provided by AIDS researchers. A cursory look at reports on the science of AIDS treatment in the news and in medical journals reveals a steady impulse of rigorous scientific innovations. Although the stories about drug and vaccine research are not always coded as "breakthrough" news, they typically appear as accumulative evidence signifying scientific progress, complete with detailed tables and graphs demonstrating how the drugs or vaccines would "really" work. A virologist characterizes this situation of AIDS drug development as follows:

> We are developing drugs exactly as we did thirty years ago, and this is not going to get the job done. The drug companies and the government are just dusting off old compounds, screening them and hoping to get lucky. It's like the days right after penicillin, when drug firms were screening soil samples everywhere from the jungles of South America to the mud basin of the Yangtze River in China. This is "wildcatting" in hopes of hitting a random oil well. (Quoted in Breo, 1988, p. 28)

As such, an overall sense of scientific rigor has appeared. "Wildcatting" may not necessarily yield useful drugs or facilitate speedy trials of the drugs, but it purports to promise us that somehow the work is being done, somehow we shall all benefit from it. The story of AZT in chapter 1 serves as a keystone case of this kind of promise, even though it is coded with ambivalence. Much of the scientific work on developing treatments for HIV/AIDS is important, but to say that science is essential to the overall intervention into the crisis is not to forget that crucial cultural fantasies and political forces continue to overdetermine the practical values and theoretical paradigms in AIDS science.

Besides the attention given to the productiveness of science, there are signs of traditional and reformed coalition efforts to develop AIDS treatment. The models represented by the Community Research Initiative based in New York and Project Inform based in San Francisco are examples of such coalitions, which involve the participation of the government, the private sectors, and grass-roots activist groups. Although such efforts are a positive sign, unfortunately journalists have generally failed to acknowledge that within these organizations, AIDS community activists and workers continue to struggle to maintain a sense of autonomy in their collaboration with technomedicine and financial institutions. The activists' strategic cooperation with mainstream medicine is often viewed, naively, as their willingness to be co-opted (see, for example, Kolata, 1988f).

In addition, within the fantasy of imagining possibilities associated with "curing," an endemic argument for maintaining a paradigm of orthodox scientific purism largely originates from certain powerful factions of the scientific community (for instance, clinical research) and is echoed by the media, traditionally obsessed with the illusions of objectivity and rationality. This is most evident in the tight observation of a single drug development method in mainstream biomedicine, namely the placebo controlled, double-blinded clinical drug trials. (Chapter 3 focuses on the struggle for change in the structure of clinical research of drugs, with important implications for the prospects for AIDS treatment.) Traditional values, whatever they may be, attempt to anchor the actual practices of drug development in a way that, although not always serving the needs of PWAs seeking treatment, never fails to interface the image of a benevolent scientist working diligently in a neutral environment, uncontaminated by political or economic forces. That image continues to carry crucial power in galvanizing a logic of rational control that, according to its own terms, will hasten the discovery of a cure.

As the tales of scientific progress offered by the popular press focus on constructing a sense of a total, collective achievement, they present scientific research as largely deindividualized, decontextualized, "synonymous" work, qualities that are the magnets for a purist rationality. For instance, in the first quarter of 1989, the *Wall Street Journal* carried a two-part report entitled "AIDS: The Race for a Cure." The first part, headlined "Tracking a Killer: Merck Scientists Find a Chink in the Armor of the AIDS Virus," discusses how researchers at Merck & Co. have successfully identified a key enzyme responsible for HIV's replication (Waldholz, 1989). The discovery reveals that it may be possible to develop a drug that would inactivate the enzyme, thereby "jam[ming] the virus' reproductive machinery." The story describes the players as "the technique," "AIDS work," "big drug makers," "the findings," "the laboratories," "the whole field of drug discovery." Apart from passing comments on biographical details, the individuals involved in the research are identified only as "the team," "researchers," "scientists," or "chemists"; they are units of a rationally organized scientific endeavor. The report concludes with a comment by a pharmacologist that continues to emphasize the anonymity or "subjectlessness" of the event: "It's a first-class piece of science. . . . It's the difference between blindly trying a lot of keys in a lock, and having a picture of the inside of the lock's tumblers." The image of unlocking a mystery is regularly combined with the image of a mystic, but steadfast, force.

The second part of the report, entitled "Homing In: Science Edges Closer to Designing Drugs to Defeat AIDS Virus" (Chase, 1989), provides what was anticipated from the first. It reveals how the findings presented in the first report have helped scientists to develop a "rational design" of drugs like CD4 that are refined and target specific. Though written by a different reporter, the second article takes a similar approach to describe the discovery, coding the story with labels such as "scores of compounds," "this knowledge," "the efforts," "a whole round of efforts," "in another plan of attack," "in the next stages of refinement," "further research is needed." As in most other science reporting, these articles construct science as an anonymous and self-propelling machine that transcends specific contexts (Myers, 1990). Whereas participants exist in AIDS research (as laboratory workers and patients), the key players in medical discoveries are frequently coded as agents of a different kind: as viruses, genetic substances, and chemical compounds, or as mythic notions such as Progress, Rationality, Control, Competition. In fact, the patients who participate in scientific experiments are often written out of these typical reports of scientific progress. Once they have been employed in scientific experiments, the status of their presence may quickly become ambiguous. In other words, in the anonymity of AIDS science, as the experimental subjects appear to be narratively subordinated to the mythic images of organic life forms, machinistic operations, and rationalist strategies, they are put in a position where their autonomy is systematically occluded. As Cindy Patton puts it:

> Science needed the speech of people with AIDS and their friends in order to unlock the "mystery" of AIDS—a Nobel Prize winning task....But once science had its information it could no longer tolerate the speech of people living with AIDS. People living with AIDS wanted some information back:

When would a cure come? What would the treatment be? What would it cost? But once the disease had been wrested out of the discourse of people living with AIDS, once HIV was discovered and could be made to perform in the laboratory without the homosexual bodies, science no longer wanted to hear that discourse. (1990, p. 130)

If hyperrationalized technology is the key figure in science reporting, then such reporting does not recognize the presence of the human subjects in illness, except when they are transformed into technologically controllable subjects.[7] Under this construction of the looming presence of Technology and the "subjectless" patient is the determination of the relative durability of the image of Technology in relation to the not-so-durable AIDS patient. The overarching logic of control cannot exist without this invisible but durable technological force.

### Policing Alternative Treatments

Within the fantasy of control, any event or phenomenon that undermines the shining visibility of rationalist technology becomes distinctively constituted as an object for containment. The fantasy is enacted with an impetus to survey any nonalignment with rationality. It is thus little wonder that one of the most active points of the fantasy of control/containment is the continued problematization of any alternative forms of treatment that have proliferated in many communities affected by HIV/AIDS. In response to the agony of the slow and narrowly focused clinical trials performed by mainstream scientists, thousands of PWAs have turned to a range of alternative medicines to alleviate pain or prolong life.

Almost as quickly as the epidemic began to affect a large number of people, and as the media and the government continued to conduct scientific research with discriminatory presumptions, PWAs created an elaborate network of physicians and agencies who would provide alternative forms of treatment for AIDS. The alternative treatment movement includes at least five dimensions:

1. The network of buyers' clubs that sell unapproved drugs otherwise unavailable or too costly to PWAs. Buyers' clubs frequently import drugs from foreign countries.

2. The host of nontoxic, holistic, often non-Western, nonallopathic treatments practiced by PWAs, including acupuncture, herbs, homeo-

pathy, nutritional supplements, diet changes, mental/spiritual programs, and bodywork (massage, yoga, therapeutic touch, and so on).

3. The ongoing information network providing the latest news on potential treatments, including community pamphlets; newsletters; and organized seminars, support groups, and national conferences on holistic treatment research (see Serinus, 1990/91).

4. The noncompliance that occurs as part of the communities' response to the restrictive methods of mainstream clinical trials (see Arras, 1990; Kolata, 1988g).

5. To a certain extent, the formation of wholly alternative views of the disease, such as the challenge to the theory of HIV as the cause of AIDS (Duesberg, 1988; Root-Bernstein, 1993); the theory that AIDS is actually the advanced stage of syphilis (Coulter, 1987); and the view that "AZT is poison" (see chapter 1). Such alternative views propagate different visions of treatment (e.g., the use of typhoid vaccine to treat syphilis).

The alternative treatment movement is a form of political resistance that, through adopting a self-empowerment model of community organizing, challenges the hyperrationalized form of technology held sacred by many mainstream scientists. The restrictive control in orthodox science has in some ways intensified the AIDS communities' attempt to take control of their own medical matters. Although alternative treatments did not of course originate with the AIDS crisis, their use and the status of alternative treatment research have never been so organized.[8] What unorthodox medical practices do is suggest a different conception of the relation of the body and technomedicine. Like the discourse of dominant medical science, unorthodox medicine establishes its validity through empirical experiential evidence of those who use it, but contrary to it, such treatment offers a stunning range of methods systematically excluded by technomedicine. More important, it stresses the relative autonomy of PWAs vis-à-vis treatment, encourages self-education, and promotes a discourse of empowerment.

Increasingly, the alternative treatment movement has met so many needs that some PWAs would choose to participate in it before they would turn to mainstream treatment protocols (Serinus, 1990/91). Far from being able to consolidate its control, the restrictive practices of technomedicine have sparked a proliferation of drug searches outside of the dominant institutional setting. Alternative treatment thus represents a partial recuperation of the patients' own control of their bodies. The

mainstream media and medical institutions are sharply critical of it, however. Federal health officials have taken action to stifle the grass-roots
movement, for fear that it may promote quack medicine and profiteering
(Robbins, 1988). Frank Young, the former FDA commissioner, comments about the movement that "every time there's a desperate disease,
people try to get rich on the suffering" (quoted in Hammer, 1988, p. 41).
The profit motive, always the underlying motive for official, "reputable"
AIDS research, is suddenly deemed problematic and thus must be
controlled.

Likewise, the mainstream press cannot seem to evaluate the significance of the alternative treatment movement without situating it in the
ideological framework of "official medicine." The reporting of health
fraud is an important task, provided that sufficiently specific information
on a case-by-case basis is clearly identified, thereby avoiding commentaries that would, in one stroke, condemn all forms of alternative medical
practices. However, the press reporting of the movement in the AIDS crisis has tended to devalue it simply on the grounds that it falls outside of
official medicine. No attempt is made to differentiate the mostly nontoxic forms of holistic medicine from potentially harmful substances found
in the underground market. As a whole, the movement is typically coded
as quackery, as an anarchistic/guerrilla operation. People who use alternative medicine are frequently constructed as exiles from their own society, uneducated consumers, gullible, desperate, or ignorant (Clark et al.,
1985; Geitner, 1988; Hammer, 1988; Kolata, 1988d; Robbins, 1988;
Ticer, 1985). Community-based clinics that provide vital information
and services of alternative treatment are termed "guerrilla clinics," operating in "the world of mischief and hucksterism," "spreading disinfor-
mation, panic and fear" (Monmaney et al., 1987). The buyers' clubs'
purchase and importation of drugs from foreign countries is often dra-
matized along the lines of an international criminal plot.

> In a brightly lit alley in Tokyo's Roppongi district, a veteran smuggler
> heads toward his first deal of the evening. Clutching a paper bag stuffed
> with crisp 10,000-yen notes, he enters a small pharmacy and within min-
> utes carries out twelve boxes filled with $40,000 worth of round white
> tablets, soon to be shipped to AIDS patients across America. The dealer is
> a registered nurse from Los Angeles, known as "Dextran Man" to most of
> his desperate customers. . . . It remains illegal to manufacture or sell [Dex-
> tran Sulphate] in the United States, and that has created a flourishing gray
> market that's fueled by altruism and greed. (Hammer, 1988, p. 41)

What was once viewed as a medical issue is now signified as a social and criminal concern, complete with the identification of the suspect and his background, the location of the crime, the illegal substance, the destination, and even the motive.

The systematic stigmatization of the alternative treatment movement by certain physicians, the press, insurance groups, pharmaceutical companies, and so-called consumer protection organizations has set in motion a wave of reaction from public health officials. In 1988, Robert Windom, the former assistant secretary for health of the Department of Health and Human Services, spearheaded an antifraud campaign against alternative health care specifically related to AIDS. Windom told the press, "I'm talking major league evil, like selling processed blue-green algae, ordinary pond scum, to gullible people who are suffering from AIDS and who clutch desperately at the hope that this might save them" (quoted in Robbins, 1988). Examples of extraordinarily problematic substances are often cited as an excuse for an open season of attack on all forms of alternative medicine. Similarly, ACT UP has reported that in 1989, Emprise, Inc., representing several leading insurance companies, proposed to create a blacklist of alternative AIDS treatment practitioners. It openly declared as the goals of its campaign support for insurance companies to reject claims by alternative practitioners, and the discouragement of government funding and support for clinical trials of alternative treatments (ACT UP, 1990b, p. 6). Although ACT UP and other AIDS activist groups succeeded in helping to overturn a funding request from the NIH by Emprise, ACT UP reported that the company has since turned to university sponsorship for its politically repellent campaign.

A background report created by ACT UP and distributed to participants at the Sixth International Conference on AIDS in 1990 effectively analyzes the systemic bias of official medicine against alternative treatment.[9] In the report, ACT UP argues that such discrimination threatens the freedom of choice and the lives of many PWAs who face a medical system—indeed, a medical history—that has driven them to use peripheral medicine and to self-organize. The criticism against potential health fraud created by certain underground treatment practitioners thus cannot be separated from the criticism against the larger, more systematically oppressive official medical structure.[10]

In the struggle for nonrestrictive choice for medical treatments, the decision to use alternative medicine is never easy.[11] The AIDS communities are caught between a systematically biased technomedicine preoccupied with prestige and financial gains, and a community-based network that relies on meager resources and that may, from time to time, experience confusion regarding the diversity of treatment methods and may even be subjected to exploitation by ill-motived practitioners, or to co-optation by market forces (Freund, 1982). It remains clear that no matter what form of treatment one determines to use, however, the matters of hope, courage, despair must not be separated ideologically into legal or illegal, moral or immoral. What are truly illegal and immoral, it is now clear to us, are the practices that devalue, submerge, or silence multiple approaches to health care and the diversity of political voices they make possible. As a physician comments, "The real quackery is among established drug companies, who will not allow [natural therapies] to be studied. Anything that is not a synthetic, patentable drug is ruthlessly suppressed" (quoted in Russell, 1990).

### The Political Tendencies of "Knowledge = Cure"

The disqualification of alternative forms of treatment, which is congruent with the fantasy of control/containment, constitutes one of the gravest obstacles in the overall effort to develop treatment for HIV/ AIDS. To many living in communities affected by HIV/AIDS, the pointed refusal to recognize the potential usefulness of alternative treatment methods has compounded their feeling of rejection by society: their effort to diversify the possibilities for healing, even as these methods carry a certain level of risk, is viewed by society as one more feature of their supposed deviancy. But it has also galvanized more systematic and more accurate delivery and monitoring of treatment information in those communities, leading to the professional crosschecking of medical opinions, the results of which are made available to PWAs in community newsletters, pamphlets, fact sheets, and regular information update meetings. Knowledge, it has been recognized, is no longer the monopoly of mainstream science. This community belief in the usefulness and power of knowledge/information, however, duplicates a broader, more endemic discourse that has been a highly visible feature of the popular lexicon of AIDS for many years, a discourse articulated in a peculiar injunction: "Knowledge = Cure."

This injunction carries a peculiar power not only as metaphor, but more importantly as a statement embraced by the communities struggling to make sense of the volume of AIDS treatment information (concerning both mainstream and alternative medicine). The general belief that curing AIDS remains a daunting task has led to the popular embrace of knowledge—the definition of which remains ambiguous—thought to be able to help prevent the further spread of the epidemic. But in what practical or imaginative framework can we say that knowledge will bring about a cure, at the very moment of our realization that curing is likely to be impossible? How does this injunction of "Knowledge = Cure" interface with the contention "AIDS is invariably fatal" already widely articulated in the fantasy of morbidity? Does *all* knowledge implicate a space that negates the morbid condition of an "invariable fatality"? If these questions point out the excessiveness of this metaphoric injunction—its multiple meanings—then the problem is how to decipher the variegated discursive contexts in which a certain type of knowledge is upheld in relation to a certain imagining of the curability of AIDS (within both the fantasy of control/containment and the fantasy of morbidity) and to observe their possible political and social effects.

Researchers and experts (including community ones) started issuing the advice that "Knowledge = Cure" almost as soon as the epidemic began, reflecting a typical rationalist public educational effort that advocates "getting the facts" as the sure shield against contracting the disease. The British government's AIDS education campaign, captured in the slogan "Don't Die of Ignorance," seems to derive from such rationalist logic. Similarly, in the United States the former surgeon general C. Everett Koop and many physicians issued a public statement about the paramount importance of "getting the facts," which became the thesis of a public education brochure, *Understanding AIDS,* mailed to every U.S. household in June 1988.

The metaphoric power of "Knowledge = Cure" rests on the conflation of crucial distinctions regarding (1) the audience assumed to be the subjects of the injunction; (2) the types of knowledge professed; (3) the imaginative forms of "cure" that result from the acquisition of a certain type of knowledge; and (4) the possible social and political effects that "Knowledge = Cure" induces (see table 2). If these distinctions are usually hidden in the invocation of such an injunction, and if we do not recognize the overarching fantasies (morbidity/control) that hold spectacular power over the multiple formations of meanings of "Knowledge = Cure," then the injunction will insist on us a rationalist thinking that may mask its political liabilities. In other words, "Knowledge = Cure" depends on our acceptance of a certain literality, objectivity, or political neutrality, and on our acceptance of its figurative power as literal.

## Table 2. The political tendencies of "Knowledge = Cure"

| Assumed subjects | Type of knowledge | (Metaphoric) cure | Possible social and political effects |
|---|---|---|---|
| "General public" | The right to know about viral transmissibility and safer sex/drug-use practices | Shielded from infection | Sanitized education through the teaching of fear; widespread testing |
| "General public" | The right to know about homosexuality and other deviancy | Shielded from "contamination" by another kind | Homophobic fantasies and policies |
| Infected "innocent" groups | The right to know about viral transmissibility and safer sex/drug-use practices | Public sympathy; forgivable infection | Public charity efforts |
| Infected "innocent" groups | The right to know about homosexuality and other deviancy | Confirmation of an "innocent" identity | Public charity efforts; creation of "truly tragic" stories |
| Infected "guilty" groups | The obligation to know about viral transmissibility and safer sex/drug-use practices | Protect the general public from contact | Abandonment; self-condemnation |
| Infected "guilty" groups | The obligation to know about viral transmissibility and safer sex/drug-use practices | Self-empowerment | Political organizing |
| Infected "guilty" groups | The obligation to know about homosexuality and other deviancy | Probable awakening; "Gay death = cure" | Redemption/ salvation/self-policing |

A hidden rhetorical and ethical structure underlies this injunction in health education that directs different strategic cognitive associations regarding the matters of knowledge and curing at what are perceived as "high-risk" or "low-risk" groups. The ubiquitous label of a "general public" commonly denotes low-risk, uninfected, nongay, non-drug users (e.g., heterosexuals). Compacted within this label is an eager belief in its mythic wholeness; that is, a belief that the so-called high-risk groups cannot already be part of it. "Closeted" gays and bisexuals and "closeted" drug users, however, exist and give a new meaning to the label. Within the infected groups is the morally and politically motivated distinction between "innocent" and "guilty" people, whose purpose is mainly to map different fantasy structures onto these categories. In other words, there is a certain circular totality in which the contradictory fantasies of morbidity/control generate categories of victim subjects, which in turn valorize the transcendent fantasies. As Cindy Patton has made clear, one of the most virulent effects of such a distinction is the creation of the assumption that the "general public" and the "infected innocent groups" receive information because they have a *right* to know, whereas the "infected guilty groups" receive information because they have an *obligation* to know so as to protect the nonguilty groups (1990, p. 103). The acquisition of knowledge is thus studded with prejudicial assumptions.

In information-giving health education, we are usually given information about the modes of viral transmission and the different (still confusing) safer sex and safer drug-use practices. Because such information is inevitably linked to a discussion of "risk" categories and "risky people," there is almost always an accompanying subtext in health education about what one needs to "know" about certain "deviant life-styles" and their respective risks. "Health information" in the context of AIDS almost never fails to articulate deviancy with health practices, rendering knowledge itself a tool for moral judgments.

The various interpellations of categories of identities and types of knowledge are the basis upon which various metaphoric "cures" can be generated. What "cure" means in "Knowledge = Cure" becomes instantly visible in light of these identity-type and knowledge-type constructions. The productiveness of these constructions must therefore not be taken lightly, because in alliance with the fantasies of morbidity/control, they structure our social, even medical, consciousness about the whole understanding of curing.

Insofar as the "general public" and the "infected innocent groups" are concerned (see table 2), knowledge about HIV's mode of transmission, safer sex and safer drug-use habits, and "deviant" practices would acquire a distinctive relation to a body of ideas about curing in terms of "shielding," "toleration," and "confirmation," thus bearing close ties to the middlebrow notions of *secure* (free from danger) and *sure* (certainty, safety), which are linked etymologically to *cure*. "Knowledge = Cure" can thus discharge a chain of privileged social and political initiatives aimed at protecting, securing, or shielding certain "clean" identity types from infection (whose meaning, in this context, is clearly less literal than metaphoric), initiatives such as sanitized forms of health education, widespread testing, public charity promotions, the creation of hyperemotive narratives about "unfortunate" victims of AIDS, and the mobilization of homophobic fantasies. Some of these initiatives often overlap (for example, sanitized health education and the call for widespread testing, which are contaminated with homophobic rhetorics; sentimental narratives that are always heard at public charity events). In such a discursive context the most common acceptance of "Knowledge = Cure" occurs in the high-comfort zone of a (mythic) insulation from bad influences. The common saying that "If science cannot yet develop a cure for AIDS, then in the meantime get the facts and protect yourself" lends enormous rhetorical charge to the fantasy of control/containment, for it hinges on the crucial semantic carrier "in the meantime," which can serve to extend temporariness ("Get educated now") to stability ("Get cured/shielded/ secured forever").

The construction of "Knowledge = Cure" in the present context has offered an equally startling injunction: "Ignorance = Disease/Death." The latter is not a mere rhetorical flip side of the former. As the performative capability of "Ignorance = Disease/Death" (featured by the British government in its "Don't Die of Ignorance" campaign in 1986) clearly lies in the defining character of ignorance—a rhetorical trope suggesting a positively inert space, a space analogous to death—we cannot regard its assumed power in the same way that "knowledge" (an entirely different trope) performs discursively. And, as "Ignorance = Disease/Death" constitutes death as its vexing component, it encourages the fantasy of morbidity, which "Knowledge = Cure" has temporarily occluded. It would be foolish to say that the two injunctions are wholly separate, however. "Knowledge = Cure," even as it actively courts the fantasy of control/ containment, *depends on* "Ignorance = Disease/Death," which performs at least three functions (see table 3). First, it recharges the morbid emotion of fear directed at every assumed group of subjects. Second, it speaks to the uninfected "high-risk" groups the durable language of gay death, thus construing "ignorance" of the risks associated with their life-styles as suicidal. Third, it rehearses the same language of gay death to the "general public," whose ignorance about HIV or about "deviant life-styles" would no longer make a significant difference within the lethal fantasy of gay genocide. Suicidal or genocidal, gay death is a permanent fixture in this injunction. I therefore suspect that the interface between "Knowledge = Cure" and "Ignorance = Disease/Death" has the effect of

Table 3. The political tendencies of "Ignorance = Disease/Death"

| Assumed subjects | Type of ignorance | Disease/death | Possible social and political effects |
|---|---|---|---|
| Uninfected "high-risk" groups | Of viral transmissibility and safer sex/drug-use practices | "AIDS is invariably fatal." | Self-policing; political organizing |
| Uninfected "high-risk" groups | Of consequence of "deviant life-styles" | AIDS, because it is a gay disease, is incurable. | Perceived as self-destruction/extinction |
| "General public" | Of viral transmissibility and safer sex/drug-use and practices | "AIDS is invariably fatal." | Demand the right of education; widespread testing |
| "General public" | Of consequence of "deviant life-styles" | AIDS, because it is a gay disease, is incurable. | Homophobic fantasies and policies |
| "General public" with "closeted" "high-risk" individuals | Of viral transmissibility, safer sex/drug-use practices, and consequence of "deviant life-styles" | AIDS, because it is a gay disease, is incurable. | Construed as "innocent" group at risk; demand the right of education; widespread testing |

enlarging the fantasy of morbidity and diminishing that of control/containment, thereby removing "curing" one mortal step from the symbolic space of life, especially of gay life, and installing such a removal as a permanent feature of such an interface.

It is thus not difficult to imagine that when "Knowledge = Cure" does speak to the "infected guilty (high-risk) groups," the metaphoric force of a "cure" associated with shielding, tolerance, confirmation, or security/ safety is pathetically weak. It is also not difficult to imagine that as the twin injunctions of "Knowledge = Cure" and "Ignorance = Disease/ Death" are directed at this group, the image of gay death is both potent and durable, allowing only a chain of morbid emotions such as guilt, abandonment, and self-condemnation, and the appearance of a benevolent call for redemption, salvation, and self-policing. The reasons for the PWA communities' embrace of "Knowledge = Cure" seem clearer in light of this analysis. Perhaps the universal desire for curing is transformed into the adoption of mainstream society's information-giving health education and public charity efforts; only after these have been adopted does the realization dawn that such efforts may create both antihomophobic and homophobic discourses. The embrace of "Knowledge = Cure" may also motivate self-empowerment in the communities, which is then transformed into political activist organizing. Activism, as PWA activist Michael Callen recognizes in his book *Surviving AIDS*, becomes the crucial middle link of this injunction: not "Knowledge = Cure," but "Knowledge = Activism = Cure." As activism and curing are linked in this way, a new force is injected into the concept of curing.

"Knowledge = Cure" indeed depends on a rhetorical implication nestled in the relation between the literal and the figural or, more accurately, in the figural *taken as* literal. This injunction appears to be the vessel of a broad, calculative rationality that attempts to establish the sanctity of rationalism itself, not by opposing itself against the figural, but by incorporating it and producing it as an effect of the literal. The political work done by "Knowledge = Cure" thus appears in the innocence of its literality. Lee Edelman has suggested:

> The AIDS epidemic [is] . . . the breeding ground for all sorts of figural associations whose virulence derives from their presentation under the aspect of literality. Indeed, one of the most disturbing features that characterizes the discourse on AIDS in America is the way in which the literal is recurrently and tendentiously produced as a figure whose figurality remains strategically occluded—a figure that thus has the potential to be used toward the most politically repressive ends. (1989, p. 302)

"Knowledge = Cure" is typical of this kind of disturbing discourse; it exemplifies the tension between figurality and literality. An education campaign that employs the equation "Knowledge = Cure" suggests an agenda that emphasizes protecting the innocent "general public" more than helping the infected or the perceived high-risk groups. Offered as literal rationality, "Knowledge = Cure" projects a naive and dangerous view that at its best raises a limited awareness of self-defense against risky behavior and even provokes political action, and at its worst reinstalls the fantasy of (gay) doom. In this way, the fantasy of control/containment appears to be something of an effect of the fantasy of morbidity.

## Summary

The two ruling structures of fantasies of AIDS in our culture are organic vectors of contradictions that have helped establish the stable definitions of AIDS as both curable and incurable. The whole question of "curing AIDS" is overdetermined by the two fantasies of morbidity and containment. Morbid fantasies of course titillate containment fantasies, and in this mutual seduction we revisit the lethal discourse that links the durable image of gay death with the emerging definitions of "curing AIDS." For medical science and the media, the focus on HIV as a prime image of a constitutive paradigm for virtually *all* understanding of AIDS and for struggling with treatment issues is among other things testimony to the power of, and the fascination with, the idea of death. In contemporary gay cultures, such a fascination with death is often viewed as an indelible mark in the specific redefinition of homosexuality since 1981.

The powerful resistance to the possibility that HIV is not uniformly and universally fatal, that the bodies of PWAs are not uniformly and universally objects of disintegration, that not every PWA is crazy about becoming the subject of scientific experiments, that not all forms and practices of alternative treatment methods are useless, and that "health education" is not always politically or culturally just education reveals to all of us, especially to gay people, an excruciatingly adamant imagination that is attempting to remove the people most affected by, and most visible in, the AIDS crisis from the spaces of life, living, safety, compassion, and power—and ultimately from the space of being "cured."

The double fantasies of morbidity/containment have authored a series of discursive pairings that are becoming basic to the modern cultural organization of the idea of an "AIDS cure": prominence/imminence, horror/hope, guilt/innocence, obligation/right, face/body, alternative/mainstream, excess/restoration, death counting/survival counting, madness/rationality, Fall/Redemption, ignorance/knowledge, extinction/survival, gay/nongay. These pairings have been particularly evident in the media representations of AIDS treatment issues.

Underlying these developments is a structuring principle with a profound influence on the cultural desire for, and the scientific protocol to develop, an "AIDS cure": the principle of timing. Temporality has emerged as a figure that mediates between the fantasies of morbidity/containment, beyond the articulation of the lethal contention that "AIDS is invariably fatal," beyond the malicious promise of gay genocide, and beyond the phantasmic prospect of a "cure" based on the timely acquisition of "knowledge." The questions provoked by such temporal modalities as now/later, has been/is going to, prominent/imminent, and prospect/promise have captured the attention of the very social institutions and power centers involved in the work of "curing AIDS," including the institutional bodies (such as the FDA) aimed at regulating the "flow" of medical treatments for HIV diseases, and the scientific work devoted to theorizing the mechanism of HIV infection in temporal terms. Discussions of the curability/incurability of AIDS cannot afford to overlook the strategic figure of time.

# 3 Temporality and the Politics of AIDS Science; or, How to Kill Time in an Epidemic

[The medical] sign, as opposed to the symptom, belongs to the field of the intelligible: by shifting from symptom to sign, the medical sign compels a mastery of time, a mastery of the disease as duration; here we recognize the very principle of Hippocratic medicine; to the very degree that it is constituted in order to master the time of the disease, the medical sign has a triple value, or a triple function; it is anamnestic, it says what has happened; it is prognostic, it says what will happen; and it is diagnostic, it says what is happening.

Roland Barthes, "Semiology and Medicine"

The biologic-scientific brontosaurus, if it is to be effective, must pass through the field of successive interrogations, according to its own rules and its own tempo, in which each stage of progress is the source of a subsequent interrogation; "immediate" medical benefits are always accidental.

Jacques Leibowitch, *A Strange Virus of Unknown Origin*

Time isn't the only thing the FDA is killing.

ACT UP poster

Time penetrates the body and with it all the meticulous controls of power.

Michel Foucault, *The Birth of the Clinic*

Every epidemic has a temporal language, a set of narratives about the disease's origin or cause, its development in time (and space), and a network of material practices by which it can be controlled according to past and future technologies. Modern biomedical science offers us an official collective "history" of an epidemic. This history, however, belongs to the field of the intelligible: as Roland Barthes has suggested, by shifting from disease to discourse, medicine compels "a mastery of time, a mastery of the disease as duration." By considering the AIDS epidemic as a temporal discourse, I hope in this chapter to illuminate a key structuring regime of knowledge that has been organized around the AIDS treatment discourse. How fast is the epidemic spreading? How quickly does information about it require updating? How quickly can the cause of illness be identified? For an infectious disease such as AIDS, how long does it take for symptoms to appear? What is the patient's possible length of survival? How quickly can the government and the medical system respond to the needs of patients? How long will funding allocation last? How quickly can a "cure" be found?

AIDS now exists largely in time: in the definitions of the life cycle and incubation period of the virus; in the categorization of the stages of illness for the patients; in the rate of the body's decay; in the principle of the phases of drug development; in the "period of efficacy" of a treatment method or a drug; in the "speed" of the drug review process; in the timeliness of responses from the government and the media, and so on. The consciousness of AIDS science is in many ways the consciousness of a set of time-oriented images and narratives.

As I have argued in the foregoing chapters, the problematic focus on "searching for a cure for AIDS" by mainstream biomedical scientists (subsequently echoed by the popular press) arises from a paradox: AIDS is simultaneously "incurable" and "curable." The former is rooted in the supposition that AIDS is "invariably fatal." The latter arises from the much more specialized professional worlds of scientists, pharmaceutical companies, information-based health education, and the regulatory bodies of the government. Their faith lies in the curative power of technomedicine, based on high standards of scientific objectivity and regulations. This paradox of the curability/incurabilityof AIDS therefore is not necessarily produced by AIDS scientists; it is rooted in the much broader linguistic, political, and fantasy terrain surrounding the epidemic, where the widespread, if not endemic, perception of AIDS has consistently fluctuated between the rhetorics of hope/hopelessness, death/salvation, body/antibody.

This paradox has also commanded contradictory perceptions of time. The fatalistic view turns time into a matter of urgency. Time is measured against a heightened sense of eventuality. Death, especially hastened death, commands a shortened sense of time. Time is bereft of its meaning; its content is reduced to its intensity, that is, an intensity of the present. In contrast, the perception of the curability of AIDS turns time into a highly productive discourse. As the emphasis is shifted to the scientific and commercial arenas, professionalism, prestige, and profiteerism (along with genuine humanitarian concern) reign. Quite literally, time becomes a field of management, something to administer. The "mastery of time, a mastery of the disease as duration," as Barthes says, thus appears to be central to the discourse of curing AIDS.

How does modern biomedicine's "mastery of time, mastery of disease as duration" become a structural logic in its practices in the United States, particularly in the ways the body with HIV conditions is conceived as temporal images in biomedical and popular discourses, and in the practices of the clinical drug trials enterprise? How does biomedicine anchor itself in a set of temporal guidelines that would, according to its own logic, produce and expedite drug treatments for AIDS? How do virological and clinical inventions such as the "HIV in time" and the "body in time" act as crucial codes that guide the programmatic logic of treatment research? If we could unpack the various modalities of time that seem to structure the AIDS scientific work, we would lay bare a major framework of knowledge that constructs the scientific subject of experimentation, in the current context of the AIDS patients' and AIDS activists' struggle over health care and survival.

I do not intend to revive archaic theories of time.[1] Rather, my response is to the discursive trajectory of AIDS that has clearly been structured around various temporal modalities. Ways of timing, rather than ways of seeing/spacing, are what seem to lend powerful authority to the mainstream biomedical agenda for AIDS.

## Split Profiles: Temporalities in Clinical and Virological AIDS

Donna Haraway argues that medical science has created a "barely contained and inharmonious heterogeneity" and that the heterogeneous discourses overlap and create "condensed contestations for meanings and practices" (1989, p. 3). Biomedical constructions of AIDS have indeed emerged as fractured narratives, usually manifest in endless quarrels among scientists. One such ongoing dispute asks why the disease progresses slowly for some individuals and more quickly for others. What is the presumed scientific logic behind HIV's infectivity? How does the presumed temporal "behavior" of HIV affect the scientists' conception of a cure for AIDS? Competing scientific theories and models have been enacted to explain the correlations among viral infectivity, immunity strength, and the emergence of symptoms. Although most scientists generally agree on specific methods for measuring each of these categories—such as monitoring the rate of activity of the molecular and genetic components of HIV for measuring viral infectivity, T4-cell count for measuring immunity strength, the number of opportunistic infections for measuring symptoms—they have not agreed on "the course of action" of the virus. The debate has emerged, among other places, between clinical medicine and genetic virology. Each of these branches of biomedicine postulates a different temporal logic regarding the development of AIDS in the body. What is most peculiar is the way their different time lines seem to build upon a rather unified cultural assumption about what it means to be infected with HIV. In the following discussion, I examine two theories and their underlying temporal logics, representing these two branches of biomedicine. The theories reflect two fairly dominant views within AIDS biomedical research around the most formative years of the AIDS treatment discourse (roughly between 1987 and 1992).

In 1988, Robert Redfield and Donald Burke of the Walter Reed Army Institute of Research in Washington, D.C., set out to explain the clinical progression of AIDS. They developed a scheme known as the Walter Reed classification system, which could plot successive stages of infection. Under this scheme, patients could be classified and managed according to their stage of infection. The two researchers postulated that, as the disease progressed, the patient moved through six stages, from initial exposure to HIV (stage 1) to systemic immune dysfunction (stage 6). A linear course of infectivity was thus established. To support their theory, they presented the result of their study of a young male patient by tracking his T4-cell concentration during the course of his illness.

> About three months after sexual exposure to HIV the patient tested positive for the virus; his T4-cell count dropped and then rebounded, presumably because his immune system temporarily controlled the infection. He developed chronic lymphadenopathy at nine months and, at 51 months, after a long, slow decline in his T4-cell count (by 36 months it was chronically below 400), exhibited chronic, subtle abnormalities of delayed hypersensitivity. He displayed persistent anergy (the complete absence of delayed hypersensitivity) at 63 months, when he developed thrush and oral hairy leukoplakia, a tongue infection. Less than a year later he was besieged by opportunistic infections, including cytomegalovirus infection, which made him blind. He died at 83 months. (Redfield and Burke, 1988, p. 94)

They concluded that the patient's disease "followed a typical course." Clearly, the dynamics of his clinical condition were reduced to a calendar, constructed in an impeccably detached language. This transformation of a person into no more than an experimental subject, a body into no more than a chart, allowed Redfield and Burke to confirm authoritatively the value of their scheme:

The system has made it possible to show that most people infected with HIV follow about the same basic course and do indeed move from stage to stage. The notion that genetic variation in the virus or distinctive features of the patients are the crucial factors influencing the disease course *has now fallen by the wayside.* (P. 97; emphasis added)

Elsewhere in their conclusion, the scientists evoked an image—literally a graph—of what they called "the balance of power" between HIV and the immune system as they shift during the course of infection (p. 97). Coded in multicolored lines and shades, the graph staged the drama of a warlike negotiation, the pushing and tugging of power between the virus and the immune system that led to eventual victory by the virus. At this point, Redfield and Burke established that "HIV then replicated wildly, killing the remaining T4 cells and hence any vestiges of immune defense" (p. 97). Throughout this whole drama, there is no indication of the individual's living through the disease. The logic of linearity thus lent discursive authority to a fatalistic view of the disease, a view that had already gained ground in virtually every discursive construction of AIDS, leaving no space for the consideration of variations in individual reaction to the virus.[2]

Molecular and genetic virologists, however, have postulated a genetically based view of the virus, focusing on the construction of the "life cycle" of the virus and its genetic makeup, which allow it to grow and to recycle across time. William Haseltine of the Dana-Farber Cancer Institute and Harvard Medical School and Flossie Wong-Staal of the National Cancer Institute, two of the most prominent AIDS scientists in the United States, saw a potential for the endless perpetuation of the virus through its reproduction from cell to cell, patient to patient (Haseltine and Wong-Staal, 1988).

Their explanation of the course of infection was grounded in two related models: the cyclical replication of the virus (commonly known as the virus's life cycle) and the interactive character of the genetic components of the virus. The growth of the virus was thought to exhibit six stages of development, from the binding between the virus's outer coat and the membrane of a host cell through the various stages of transcription of the virus's genetic components. The final stage occurred when the viral proteins were reassembled into new complete particles (pp. 52-53). This life cycle theory postulated that the viral development did not stop at the sixth stage. At least in the context of genetic virology, there could be no endpoint to the virus's growth. Like hot air in a closed container, the reassembled viral particle reentered the cycle of genetic replication at the site of a new host cell. Time ran circularly. On this basis the widely adopted methodology of AIDS treatment was created: the design of "target drugs" for each specific stage of infection, often accompanied by pictorial descriptions of the HIV life cycle and the rational approach to treatment found in the popular press and in scientific publications (see fig. 6).

The genetic virologists had also postulated that an elaborate set of genetic controls determined whether the virus's cycle of replication would be played out and how fast it would proceed (p. 55). The HIV genome was thought to possess three major genes (named tat, rev, and nef) that regulated the rate of the virus's action. Two regulators sped up protein synthesis, and the third repressed it, forming an interactive network of complex control. The rate of infection thus depended on the counteractive pulses of the different genes. This genetic model matched the life cycle model in that both emphasized circularity and interactivity, a nonlinear temporal structure.

Together, clinical medicine and genetic virology constructed a fairly unified spectacle of HIV infectivity: whereas the virus was capable of reproducing itself in endless cycles, the person with the virus was doomed to a linear and eventual demise. It was within this difference in temporal order that the deep horror of AIDS was implied: the horror of a guaranteed death sentence for the infected individual, compounded by the horror of HIV as an agent capable of living on, leaping from one victim to another, abandoning them after using them as the breeding ground for more of its own. Within this structure, certain oppressive metaphors emerged in the popular consciousness that are now commonly used to characterize the experience of living with AIDS: the metaphors that people with AIDS are "time bombs" (as if saying, "They are going to die at any moment") and that they live on "borrowed time" (as if saying, "They should be dead by now"). The popular press has gravitated toward such constructions, and the typical narrative of time bombs and borrowed time associated with PWAs or HIV constructs a cynical view that any attempt to try to stay alive would only be "postponing the inevitable." In journalist Marilyn Chase's (1988a) report in the *Wall Street Journal*, people with AIDS are termed "people . . . living on death row," "all of them people who were dying," "people immobilized by their terror" (p. 1). Fatalism, she seems to suggest, is what they should passively accept, not struggle against. She also says, typically, "Medical

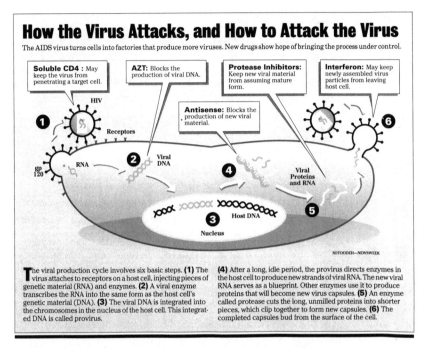

Figure 6. Tailor-made treatment relies on a one-to-one matching of HIV's points of vulnerability and different drugs' supposed antiviral functions. Reprinted with permission from *Newsweek,* June 25, 1990, p. 22.

science is in a race against time" (Chase, 1988a, p. 1). In this way, natural time eludes intervention, when in fact time itself is a social construction. The virus as bomb is both the constantly ticking threat of life and the merciful master who temporarily preserves life but who will eventually terminate it at its own "natural" will.

Such temporal images and narratives in AIDS science are in some ways cultural artifacts invoked, woven into, and even legitimized by the scientific practices already imbued with a temporal structure. As we have seen, the body in illness exists as an image and narrative of time. It also plunges into the timetable of institutional technomedicine, which constructs—and regulates—the possibility of curing according to its own temporalities. Put another way, AIDS is doubly articulated in time: the scientific texts of AIDS tell time, and they do so in the larger context of institutional temporalities. Such institutional temporalities are most visible in the practices of the clinical drug trial.

## The FDA and the Discourse of "Expediency"

In writing about the evolution of AIDS treatment activism, Paula Treichler (1991) reminds us that contemporary medical sciences embrace the technoethics of organized research conducted in the industrial-regulatory milieu. Orthodox institutional practices in the search for AIDS treatment are increasingly viewed as inappropriate in the face of the AIDS crisis, however. Since 1987, a "reform" of medical research has been under way, carrying with it the potential to transform the practices of clinical drug trials, particularly their pace. Everyone, it seems, was anxious for the quick release of drugs, including Wall Street and church leaders. What were the historical conditions of possibility out of which this reform of clinical trial practices emerged? How was the reform organized by the medical apparatuses, institutionally as well as discursively? Most important, how did this reform, constructed with a new temporality, improve access to new drugs for AIDS? Or did it?

The history of the development of the Public Health Service (PHS), of which the National Institutes of Health (NIH), the Food and Drug Administration (FDA), and the Centers for Disease Control (CDC) are a part, reveals two biases that were to affect treatment care for AIDS significantly. First, since the establishment of the Food and Drugs Act in 1906 (a response to public concern about the hazards and abuse associated with patented medicine and food), regulation had been effectively separated from health care. During the next sixty years, more and more legislative measures were introduced regarding the health care system, most notably the Food, Drug, and Cosmetic Act of 1938 and the Kefauver Amendment of 1962. The idea of sound regulation was accepted as the universal solution to the problems of abuse found in the history of medical experimentation involving human subjects (such as the Tuskegee Syphilis Study) and to other massive tragedies resulting from the use of unsafe drugs (such as the Elixir Sulfanilamide disaster in 1937 and the Thalidomide incident in the early 1960s).[3] Thus, to have health care was first to call for a reform of regulation; the matter of health became a way of governing. Under the FDA, "proof of safety and efficacy" became the master code for the approval, licensing, and marketing of any health-related products. The regulatory imperative was closely associated with the need for "good science." A section of the Kefauver Amendment reads:

> If there is a lack of substantial evidence that the drug will have the effect it purports or is represented to have under the conditions of use prescribed,

recommended or suggested in the proposed labeling thereof . . . [the secretary of health and human services] shall issue an order refusing to approve the application. . . . The term "substantial evidence" means evidence consisting of adequate and well-controlled investigations, including clinical investigations, by experts qualified by scientific training and experience to evaluate the effectiveness of the drug involved. (Cited in ACT UP, 1988, p. 7)

Regulatory medicine emerged in conjunction with the rise of corporate power in the medical field (particularly during the New Deal era), which had successfully lobbied for the independence and autonomy of pharmaceutical companies in their marketing strategies (for instance, in the pricing and distribution of drugs). Scientific regulation and market economics thus became the vital determinants of public health care.

The second bias that would affect AIDS treatment is that following the separation of regulation from health care came the separation of basic research from health care. As Sandra Panem (1988) has suggested, the evolution of contemporary public health institutions has reflected a direct interest in the critical separation between fundamental scientific efforts and clinical services.[4] The domination of basic research in the medical field was also a result of direct federal involvement through authorizing federal grant funds for basic research. What occurred was the restructuring, in a precise historical context, of the discourse of the "liberation of medicine": medical truth was defined more and more in institutional and scientific terms, and the priority of research was to be separated vigilantly from that of treatment, in conception as well as in practice. The liberation discourse emerged not only out of political opportunism (the year of the enactment of the Kefauver Amendment, 1962, was an election year), but also out of a fidelity to a technoethics marshaled against ignorance (associated with the lay public), bewilderment (associated with the patient), profiteerism (associated with the quack doctors), and anything else that might obscure the scientific pursuit of truth.

From these historical conditions—the separation of regulation and research from health care—the current practice of clinical drug trials emerged. Scientists assure us that controlled clinical trials are the fastest way to determine if a given therapy exerts the desired therapeutic effect, that no other method accomplishes this end as rapidly and effectively (see, for example, Myers and La Montagnier, 1987). Expediency is offered up as the key quality of the clinical trials. A language of temporality is now attached to the clinical trials process.

The fundamental act in the design of a clinical trial is to establish a temporal logic. Before measurement can take place, before a substance can be "proven" useful or not, sufficient time must be given to the subject's body to assimilate or react to the substance. The rather primitive notion that "you have to allow time for the subjects to react to the drug" is made into official dogma: The longer the trial takes, the better it proves the safety and efficacy of the drug. A "controlled" experiment never constructs certain variables without simultaneously measuring those variables against time. Even the most austere forms of scientific expression, such as the "Graph" and the "Chart," report the interactions of various elements with time, that important "t" factor. In the practice of clinical trials, this temporal imperative is expressed in the typical three-phase structure: phase 1 studies establish the safety of the drug; phase 2 studies conduct highly controlled double-blinded placebo trials to determine the drug's efficacy; phase 3 studies provide additional data on drug efficacy, set proper dosages, and develop sufficient safety information to establish the drug's risk-benefit ratio.

Moreover, in order to further secure time as the indispensable arbiter of a drug's safety and efficacy, scientists are also concerned with the status of the subject's conditions of illness, within the already created *interpretive* framework regarding clinical knowledge about the disease. Specifically, an understanding of where the subject falls in the preconceived time line of the disease at the time of the experiment has to be sought, because researchers argue that it figures into the overall determination of the drug's efficacy (Young, 1989). The question of "When can the drug be determined as useful to a patient?" does not merely depend on "How long has the patient been participating in the trial and taking the drug?" It is also implicated within another more fundamental question: "How long has the patient been ill?" In the case of AIDS, the longer the patient has been ill, the more "pathological" is the individual (measured in terms of symptoms), hence the more "ideal" an experimental subject the individual becomes. This explains why there are few clinical trials designed for individuals in the early stages of their illness (that is, when they are asymptomatic), because they are perceived as not having sufficiently definable clinical conditions and are therefore not ideal for scientists to determine the usefulness of a drug based on their clinical manifestations. In effect, they are "too early" for the experimental drug in the calculated time line of the experiment.

The design for the trial therefore may emerge not from a set of independent scientific guidelines but from the preconceived time map of the disease: the body is situated within the disease, the disease in a specific time line, and this time line in the general plan of the treatment apparatuses. If the clinical trial is to produce an effective treatment, it must first construct and legitimize this time map. Arguably, without the scientific discourses that detail the life span of diseases and their temporal schedules, the discourse of the clinical trial would not be complete.

The clinical trial has been a point of direct conflict in the struggle for AIDS treatment (Edgar and Rothman, 1991, 1992; Erni, 1992b; Treichler, 1991). After a decade of trials, the major point of protest from AIDS activists and physicians against them is still the problem of timing.[5] AIDS activists have expressed their frustration toward the FDA's lengthy trial processes. Protests are sometimes deliberately designed around the theme of timing, and activists have created public awareness about it. They have disrupted speeches by holding up their watches with alarms ringing in order to remind the officials that people with AIDS are tired of waiting or simply cannot wait. One ACT UP poster states: "Time isn't the only thing the FDA is killing," implying that the consciousness of the struggles with the FDA is inseparable from the consciousness of time, that the killing of time equals the killing of people, and pointing out that the allowed loss of time is criminal, for it means the loss of life. These political actions underscore the tyranny of time that the FDA has imposed on people with AIDS. Rather fundamentally, the struggle for AIDS treatment has to be won over time: over the restructuring of the time line and timeliness of research.

Since 1987, the FDA has attempted to respond to the public pressure by implementing a series of changes to the clinical trials process. According to FDA spokespersons, these changes would revolutionize the history of medical treatment by substantially expediting the drug review process (see Graham, 1991; Nightingale, 1989; F. Young, 1988). In 1987, in response to ongoing protests by various AIDS activist groups, the FDA issued new regulations that would permit the use and marketing of investigational new drugs while still in clinical trials (F. Young, 1988). The new rules sparked a whole new consciousness about medical research, a new discourse of expediency that captured the attention of the press and medical journals. The press helped medicine speak a new language of time:

"U.S. Studies Ways to Speed Up Drugs for Seriously Ill" (*New York Times*, August 7, 1988)

"U.S. Looking for Short Cuts to Speed Drug Approval" (*Nature*, August 18, 1988)

"FDA Looks to Speed Up Drug Approval Process" (*Science*, September 16, 1988)

"FDA Offers Plan to Speed Process of Drug Approval" (*Boston Globe*, October 20, 1988)

"Drug Firms Hope FDA Broadens Plan to Speed Approval of Some Medicine" (*Wall Street Journal*, October 21, 1988)

"Cutting Red Tape to Save Lives: The FDA Vows to Speed Up Approval of Breakthrough Drugs" (*Time*, October 31, 1988)

"FDA Seeks Swifter Approval of Drugs for Some Life-threatening or Debilitating Diseases" (*Journal of American Medical Association*, November 25, 1988)

"Panel Seeks to Streamline FDA for Cancer and AIDS Drugs" (*New York Times*, January 5, 1989)

"FDA Acts to Speed Approval of Drugs" (*New York Times*, February 21, 1989)

"Regulatory Update: The FDA Speeds Up Hope for the Desperately Ill and Dying" (*American Business Law Journal*, Fall 1989)

"At Last, Quicker Access to AIDS Drugs" (*Newsweek*, July 10, 1989)

"Quick Release of AIDS Drugs" (*Science*, July 28, 1989)

"A Fast Track for Drugs" (*The Economist*, August 12, 1989)

"How the AIDS Crisis Made Drug Regulators Speed Up" (*New York Times*, September 24, 1989)

"Speed Testing: AIDS Drugs in the Field" (*New York Newsday*, December 1989)

"U.S. Moves to Help Critically Ill Get New AIDS Drugs" (*Wall Street Journal*, March 21, 1990)

"Cutting the Red Tape on AIDS Drugs" (*Business Week*, February 25, 1991)

However simplistic these announcements may be, they have helped to reestablish a new faith in the drug approval process. Even hope can be expedited in the new language of time spoken by technomedicine. This new discourse of expediency began when the FDA announced its Treatment Investigational New Drug (IND) program in 1987. What was new

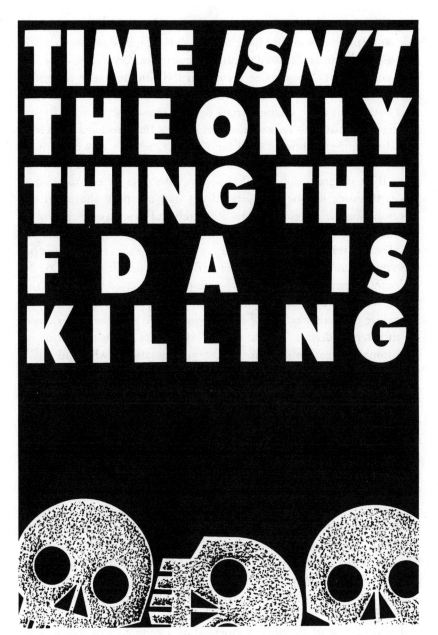

Figure 7. The consciousness of the struggles with the FDA is inseparable from the consciousness of time. The killing of time equals the killing of people. Reprinted with permission from Douglas Crimp and Adam Rolston, *AIDS Demo Graphics*, p. 77.

about the program was that it proposed that a drug might be made available, sometimes as soon as phase 2 of the clinical trial was completed, as long as sufficient data existed to prove the drug's safety and efficacy. But the issuance of the drug under Treatment IND did not mean the end of the trial. In fact, the new regulations made authorization of a Treatment IND contingent upon ongoing trials beyond phase 2. It was hardly surprising that under this reform, the trial process that preceded the release of a drug under Treatment IND (and after its release) was much more aggressively monitored than before. AIDS activists argued that the Treatment IND program did not change the FDA's restricted standard of proof; the time it took to release drugs had not been shortened (see "Deciphering the System," 1991; "Research and Regulation," 1988).

Specific criteria must be met for the Treatment IND to be approved by the FDA.[6] In the new procedure's first year, the agency released only one experimental drug, trimetrexate, for early use by people with AIDS. But under tight restrictions, only eighty-nine people received the drug in that year ("Research and Regulation," 1988, p. 3), presumably because the procedure restricted the release of the drug only to those with "serious or life-threatening disease." In the case of AIDS, that means the full-blown symptomatic stage; those who were asymptomatic or who had AIDS-related conditions were therefore excluded. Moreover, under the new procedure, pharmaceutical companies were not required to apply for Treatment INDs, and the agency did not provide sufficient incentive for them to do so. In fact, the lack of liability protection and the ambiguity of the standards made most companies reluctant to submit applications, for fear that a denial could set approval back one or more years. During the first year, only four company requests were made for Treatment INDs, three of which were denied. The situation was further compounded by problems the new regulations had failed to consider, such as the delay of trials because of insufficient staffing (Boffey, 1988a, 1988c) and the extensive bureaucratic procedures for disseminating critical treatment information to physicians and the public (Kolata, 1990a; Panem, 1988, pp. 110-17). In the *Final Report of the Presidential Commission on the Human Immunodeficiency Virus Epidemic* (Presidential Commission, 1988), these new rules were termed a drastic failure.

The discourse of expediency emerged as a campaign of compassion, and, as public criticism grew, it quickly retreated to highly defensive rhetoric and sometimes to outright denial. In announcing the new rules, FDA commissioner Frank Young said, "I've seen a lot of folks who are suffering, and I want those people who have either cancer or AIDS to know that this agency has a heart as well as mind" (cited in Silver, 1988). On another occasion, Young commented on his own experience as a physician:

> When I was caring for patients, people would occasionally come to me who had a spouse or child suffering from some untreatable disease or who were themselves desperately ill. They'd ask my help in obtaining some promising but still experimental treatment . . . I'd have to explain that the controlled clinical trials . . . were necessary, even though they took precious time. . . . The memory of such anguish and hopelessness still haunts me, and now our new regulations offer the promise of hope, acknowledging that there are times when an experimental drug shows such promise that it seems unethical and even cruel to withhold it from desperate patients. (Cited in Breo, 1988, p. 14)

In July 1988, when Young announced that the FDA would permit the importation of unapproved drugs from abroad for personal use, he offered the same sympathetic prose: "There is such a degree of desperation, and people are going to die, that I'm not going to be the Commissioner that robs them of hope" (cited in Boffey, 1988d). Young's comments were peculiarly ironic, however, for at the same time the press had been issuing an outpouring of criticism from AIDS activists, physicians, and congressional health leaders that the FDA's new rules had failed to produce new drugs for AIDS and that the agency that championed itself as the guardian against false hope had offered the public exactly that ("AIDS and 1962," 1988; Boffey, 1988b; "New Ideas," 1988). The FDA's "gentle reform," when reexamined, masked a harsh violation of the patient's basic rights to drug access and treatment.

Frank Young rebutted criticisms first by denial and then by numerical speculation. In an interview, he replied to the press: "We can't approve something that isn't there. . . . I think we'll see a substantial number of drugs coming through for AIDS in the future" (quoted in Boffey, 1988b). At that time, according to various industry reports, at least nine AIDS-related drugs were approaching the final phase of human testing (ibid.). A week later in a Senate hearing, Young issued a statistical projection that, "based on past experience with other experimental drugs," current trials would not yield more than one or two drugs by 1991 that would be useful for treating AIDS (Boffey, 1988f). The former FDA commissioner's optimistic rhetoric and compassionate tone of a year earlier had changed to denial and pessimism.

Worse still, a year later, when he testified to the National Committee to Review Current Procedures for Approval of New Drugs for Cancer and AIDS, he responded to critics of the agency and its collapsing new rules by regressing to the most compulsively repeated defense:

> While patients in trials generally get excellent medical care related to the disease or condition under study, the primary purpose and focus of a clinical trial is to answer an important drug development question, not to be a health care delivery system. (Young, 1989)

Conservatives had also echoed this repellent view. Professor of health law George Annas (1990) maintained that experimentation could not be confused with therapy and that the FDA should not give in to political pressure that could jettison high scientific standards:

> Certification by the FDA of the safety and efficacy of drugs recognizes that the public is in no position to judge the value or usefulness of many medications and that many are dangerous and have serious side effects. . . . Furthermore, drug manufacturers have another social role: to create and sell new products. Their role is not consumer protection. (Annas, 1990, p. 191; see also Marwick, 1988)

In the midst of rising public distrust of and confusion over the politics of the FDA's conduct, Professor Annas's hard-nosed rhetoric was entirely untenable, if not downright naive. Still others attributed the problems of clinical trials to the subjects' failure to follow scientific procedures closely, and to their refusal to cooperate by lying to or cheating the researchers (see Arras, 1990; Kolata, 1988g). "Efficiency" in clinical trials thus became the moral duty of the subjects—to keep appointments, to comply with the demands of the protocols, to change "life styles" in order to accommodate science, and so on.[7]

The series of responses from the FDA and its supporters revealed that the fundamental biases of medical research had not changed. Most of all, the FDA had not in any significant way improved access, in terms of increasing the number of drugs available for PWAs, or widening the selection criteria for recruiting subjects, or streamlining the bureaucratic procedures involved in conducting research. Let me emphasize that what occurred was not a conspiracy against fast drug approval, but a whole movement in medical research that, in its specific ideological context, managed to create a new moral discourse *without* significantly altering the practices of traditional science. This movement facilitated a new ethic of research without facilitating a new system of access to treatment. The reform concealed the difference between rearranging design and access through a false association of time and change.

As long as the FDA's clinical trial design maintains a firm control of the clinical research of AIDS by absorbing itself into a singular time line or schedule (however "flexible" it may be), the prospect for improving access to drugs to treat AIDS will remain limited. The burden, it seems, will be to open up alternatives above or around this structure without completely abandoning it. One solution, as was gradually made clear, would be to attempt to implement coexisting, multiarmed research involving various degrees of drug availability and various numbers of subjects. Activists began to argue that expanding access to experimental drugs could occur when a more flexible track of clinical trials (designed to administer the experimental drugs to a large population of AIDS patients at *all* stages of their illness) was added to the traditional controlled trials carried out on a relatively small number of patients. The idea of parallel-track research was foreseen by Mathilde Krim of the American Foundation for AIDS Research (AmFAR) in 1986, subsequently adapted and advocated by Anthony Fauci of the National Institute of Allergy and Infectious Diseases in 1989, and widely endorsed by various AIDS organizations, including ACT UP/NY, Gay Men's Health Crisis, AmFAR, Project Inform, and the National Association of People with AIDS.[8]

By allowing a significantly wider access to experimental drugs to those who were previously excluded for various reasons, by properly honoring the patients' wish to receive and use the drugs, and by retaining the traditional (and limited) research model for obtaining clinical data to determine the drugs' usefulness, the parallel-track model finally offered a plan that could benefit the patients. Moreover, the plan was proposed with the stipulation that a separate advisory committee (organized by various AIDS groups, community physicians and researchers, and the drug companies) would have "full decision-making autonomy" in reviewing the progress of drug research, a committee independent of the FDA. Parallel-track research therefore provided a new vision not limited by attention to a singular time line; it added to the existing structure a second, potentially more "democratic" time line. Through such an addition—in fact, through a theory of a multiplicity of time lines—future reform of the regulation of AIDS clinical research must be carried out. The demand for a better timing of the release of drugs requires us to continue to deconstruct the temporal structures of organized clinical research and the ways that they interpellate our bodies.

## The Figure of Time: Some Theoretical Considerations

Seen in relation to time, a disease becomes exhaustively discernible, deeply implicated in the systematic calculation of the chart, the time table, the schedule. Yet time is not an empirically discernible entity but rather lies in our ways of thinking; cultural constructs create for us different forms of practices and time consciousness. "Time is scarce," we are constantly reminded by AIDS scientists and medical journalists. As I have tried to point out in this chapter, however, this profound tyranny of time arises not only from the reality of the material body but also from the pervasive, but nonetheless incomplete, articulations of time through biomedical discourses.

Foucault's early writing, especially *The Birth of the Clinic* (1975), has been central to a theoretical and political understanding of the issues of medical discourse and body politics. But the fact that Foucault is rarely discussed in the study of time and its relation to the body points to his bias toward a mode of historical analysis centered on the spatialization, not the temporalization, of the body. To be sure, we must fully embrace the significance of spatialization in considering medical practices, but we need to ask, borrowing from Foucault's theoretical strength, what fundamental relation medical knowledge has to the spatialization of the body, other than the relation with the act of the gaze. Is there not a positive temporal dimension to the body, corresponding to its spatial dimension? Does the presence of disease in the body, that "whole dark underside of the body" described by Foucault, objectified by the reductive discourses of the doctor and the medical researcher, compel a discourse of endless depth and palpitation? I am suggesting, simply, that the language of spatialization is insufficient for gaining a secure footing upon medical matters; a "rational" discourse of the body in medicine also requires a language of temporality.[9]

If clinical medicine represented a move, as Foucault (1975, p. xviii) has suggested, from the doctor's asking, "What is the matter with you?" to "Where does it hurt?" is it not probable to imagine the discourse quickly shifting to: "How long has it been hurting?" "When did it last hurt?" "How far apart does it hurt?" Moving from the domain of diagnosis to that of prescription, is there not an elaboration of the whole discourse by the doctor's administration of drugs, designed with an underlying cyclical regularity? If we accept that modern technomedicine has moved rapidly toward the temporalization of the body, as in the case of

AIDS, we may then ask what time line, whose time line, anchors the power relations that determine the possibilities of treatment.

Just as the rejuvenation of medical perception in the late seventeenth century was based on an empiricism constructed by the organization of the gaze, modern medical perception seems to have been articulated through the organization of the "chart." Not only the chart that records the daily or hourly course of illness of the patient, but the chart that regulates the flow of the research act, the chronological steps of the experimentation, the time taken to disseminate research findings to the public, and all the cultural clocks that purport to tell us the time to worry, to sign up as experimental subjects, to get off when "time runs out." The cultural time tables of science document and justify the hard necessity of science's own temporal agendas.

In thinking through the concept of time and its relations to the body, one might discover three different operations. The concept of time sense provides us with a way of understanding the discursive arrangement that holds up the body as a scientifically quantifiable and thus potentially treatable entity (the "chart" that plots the course of infection being the obvious example). In distinction, the concept of tempo points to the felt sense of the time of the disease, the material experience of its development. Finally, the concept of temporality refers to the epistemological ordering of knowledge, delineating what may count as "useful" or "productive" time that the body can be made to offer; in short, it demarcates useful bodies from wasteful ones in the so-called larger scheme of things.

This triadic structure, which has increasingly exposed the tensions and conflicts between a technoscientific logic and lived experience, demands a historical reassessment of biomedicine. The politicized consciousness of timing/timeliness created by AIDS treatment activism has exposed the lived contradictions between how we experience and deal with our own illness in time and how we are represented in research time. Compassion, we have realized, is fragile in the face of competition, economic gain, and regulation. The anatomical disease alone cannot explain our vulnerability.

## Summary

The onset of the AIDS crisis has generally uncovered the previously hidden cultural crisis of medicine in the context of a growing conservative polity (Fox, 1988). But more narrowly, AIDS forces us to reevaluate critically the temporality of biomedical practices in their institutional context. For instance, the FDA's concern with "safety and efficacy" is, though important, not an objective independent of a disciplinary structure similar to the Taylorist ideal aimed at organizing the body temporally for the purposes of efficiency and supervision.[10] How we fight AIDS therefore becomes, in part, a question of where we are positioned on the disciplinary time lines of corporate and scientific medicine.

Currently, the public consciousness of the ever-rising death toll of AIDS and the ever-increasing number of people who will fall ill in the coming years has further eroded the already questionable status of medical judgment and has demanded a revolution over the very organization of time. What were championed as the unprejudiced practices of medicine, the "fair time" of clinical research, have been fundamentally challenged. The perpetually objectified correlations between the "timeable" and the "experimentable" in biomedicine can no longer be used for the ultimate organization of clinical research. We should not abandon experimentation once and for all, but we must break away from the tyrannical ordering of time over our bodies. We must write our own time lines (temporality), according to our individual assessment of our own conditions of health (tempo) and our collective determination of where, when, and how our bodies will be used for research (time sense). The emergence of parallel-track research and its support by community-level research efforts are signs of a popular force trying actively to reorganize this temporal politics of AIDS research.

The theoretical understanding of how the human body is circumscribed by the rhythms of experimentations and trials, the time table of treatment, the cyclical character of illness, the rhetorics of projection, and so on, can give us insight into ways of changing medical perceptions and practices. As we grapple with health care reform in the Clinton years, such a theoretical understanding will benefit us in the assessment of patient care in the changing temporal organization of medical practices. We have recently seen a shift in the medical perception of AIDS from a fatalistic model to a health management model. This shift is critically important because it stems from a drastically different understanding of the ethics, economics, and politics of time. Perhaps the time has come to discuss seriously the meanings of, the material practices associated with, and the political force in the phrase long-term survival.

# 4 Power and Ambivalence: The Conjunctural Crises of Technomedicine and AIDS Treatment Activism

SILENCE = DEATH. When I first saw this poster I believed it said "Science = Death." I had no doubt that this was what I had read. When the poster became a button, a T-shirt, the key symbol of the anarchistic resistance to a pogrom masquerading as a disease, I was sure that the slogan had been changed. . . . But the dyad silence/science was no mistake. Straight people find this slip funny. Gay people do not.

Cindy Patton, *Inventing AIDS*

We must recognize that "our" "activist" discourse is only a *mutation* of "their" "master discourses" and that its effect on them, though certain, is also always unpredictable.

Lee Edelman, "The Mirror and the Tank"

My aim in this book has been to examine the phenomenon of "curing AIDS" from the perspective of the "discursive field" in which it occurs. Any "insider's view" of AIDS treatment development offered by the agencies, organizations, or individuals associated with treatment activities—activities that include technological practices, regulatory/governmental practices, medical reports, and press coverage—is, in my view, commanded by this discursive field. The historical and structural conditions that produce "curing" as the central signifier for AIDS treatment are the real critical ground upon which the whole treatment discourse is constructed, in the specific forms and formations it has taken. I have argued that this discursive field is structured by the overall, totalizing definition of the curability/incurability of AIDS. This stable contradiction has created a sense of psychosocial paralysis in coping with the complex realities of AIDS treatment (as evident in the story of AZT), has reinscribed the bureaucratic structures most responsible for producing treatment for HIV diseases by lending support to their temporal control of the body, and even has reactivated the lethal fantasy of massive gay death articulated through the transcendental fantasies of morbidity/containment.

In the context of technomedicine, this totality created by the bifurcated terms of curability/incurability must not be seen as a paradox. At a fairly literal level, it appears that there is a causal and "natural" relationship whereby the devastating reality of AIDS (incurability/morbidity) exists in part to bolster technomedicine's curative power (curability/control). The statement "Medicine controls AIDS" appears most natural and authoritative, an assertion made possible by the prior statements about the horrific images of HIV and the AIDS body, the grim projections, and the scandal of the underground treatment movement. The seemingly contradictory perspectives of curability and incurability can now be conjoined in the most common, folklike tale of disease and disease control.

The social and symbolic power the terms of curability/incurability carry rests on a unified "totality in contradiction," a monster with two heads. Together, the terms curability and incurability are particularly provocative of a complex drama wherein the twin poles of fascination and paranoia appear as two completely compatible economies. We are fascinated, because we are offered the deep mysteries of the morbid corporeal and social dimensions. We are paranoid because this phantasmal scientific sphere simultaneously exposes the wonder and limitation of science. Fascination and paranoia are frequently what construct the most "commonsensical" ideas about medical authority. Moreover, the terms of curability/incurability are full of historical and political ramifications; they are not simply textual descriptors. They have become the "nodal points" (Laclau and Mouffe, 1985)—the discursive frontiers—for the articulation of a potentially changing political climate for technomedicine.

To grasp the historical implications and political effectiveness of the phenomenon of "curing AIDS" and its discursive field, we need to examine a problem only implicitly addressed so far in this book: the relationship between "curing AIDS" and the main social constituency with which the entire crisis has been identified—gays, particularly gay men, and the AIDS treatment activist movement. As the construct "AIDS" has been connotatively rich in its reference to (male) homosexuality from the outset, and as the whole gaying of AIDS has served to incite an a priori conception of other oppressed communities that are not made up of gay males (notably lesbians) as mirroring the constructed experiences of gay men in the crisis, one might think that an essentially uniform gay subjectivity would have appeared in the discourse of "curing AIDS." Yet nothing in the coupling of gays and AIDS within technomedical and media discourses across the fluid fantasies of morbidity/containment necessarily gives rise to a unitary gay subject. Even as the gay communities have constructed themselves around the oppositional discourses of both AIDS treatment activism and queer politics, subjectivity remains a matter to be negotiated among themselves and across the various communities within the two political movements.

An examination of the relationship between medical reform in the context of the AIDS crisis and the politics of the AIDS treatment activist movement in the discourse of "curing AIDS" can shed light on the question of the negotiating "agent," the *subject of curing*, usually (from within the paradigmatic vision of the discourse), a gay male subject. Because we cannot assume that medical reform and activist politics are always dichotomous, we cannot predict the social or political status of that subject of curing. If we understand the shifting nature of the gay subject at the present historical moment of profound changes—indeed, crisis—in technomedicine and in treatment activism, we open an important path for thinking about the question of power and hegemony at the critical frontier of queer politics.

## Legitimation through Crisis

In what ways is technomedicine redefining the sense of "crisis" it sets out to "control," based on the dominant definition of curability/incurability? Curing a disease and controlling a crisis are very different things; they construct very different patterns of signification; they mobilize very different resources. If the folklike tale of disease and disease control signifies the crisis-controlling power of technomedicine, the question is, what crisis is it responding to and controlling? Could it be that AIDS, far from being a new medical crisis, focuses what is already a preexisting crisis? Could there be a larger and deeper crisis than the immediate AIDS panic confronting biomedicine? Could it be that the present AIDS crisis arises in the midst of a general cynicism in society toward the social and political authority of a health polity based largely on orthodox technocratic medicine?

Daniel Fox, among many other medical historians and medical policy analysts, has documented a crisis of authority in public health and medicine that long preceded the AIDS crisis. He argues that a series of changes have transformed biomedical research and the U.S. health care system in general, challenging the social prestige of organized medicine.

> When the AIDS epidemic began, a profound crisis of authority was transforming the American health polity. The roots of this crisis reached back in time, some for decades, others for just a few years. They included

changes in the causes of sickness and death and, therefore, concerted efforts to adapt facilities and payment mechanisms in order to address them; ambivalence about the recent progress of medical research, reflected in slower growth in research budgets and efforts to make scientists more accountable to their financial sponsors and the media; a growing belief that individuals should take more responsibility for their own health and that public health agencies should encourage them to do so; a sense that the cost of health care was rising uncontrollably and should be contained; and an increase in the power of the private sector and of the states within the health polity. (Fox, 1988, pp. 316-17)

Health care professionals were well aware that a crisis was occurring. Fox adds, "Uncertainty about priorities, resources, and most important-ly, leadership pervaded the health polity" (p. 317). AIDS did *not* cause this pervasive sense of crisis. The crisis of authority predated AIDS and subsequently structured the current crisis.

The advent of AIDS has caused many in the health care field to reex-amine the overall conditions of public health and the practices of main-stream medicine. Back in November 1988, the Institute of Medicine issued a report entitled *The Future of Public Health* that confirmed that the public health system was "in disarray." The American Public Health Association described the report as "a terrible indictment of the current status of public health" (cited in "Nation's Public Health," 1988). The institute's panel conducted extensive hearings, made site visits to six states, and collected private testimonies. It concluded:

We have observed disorganization, weak and unstable leadership, a less-ening of professional and expert competence in leadership positions, hos-tility to public health concepts and approaches, outdated statutes, inade-quate financial support for public health activities and public health education, gaps in the data gathering and analysis that are essential to the public health functions of assessment and surveillance and lack of effec-tive links between public and private sectors for the accomplishment of public health objectives. (Cited in "Nation's Public Health," 1988, p. 12)

Again and again, reports that attempt to make sense of the future trends of health care have forced researchers to reexamine the ongoing prob-lems in the history of the system (see, for example, Enthoven, 1989; Fox, 1990a, 1990b; Rogers, 1986; Todd, 1990). The frustration of attentive citizens and consumers with orthodox medical practices has led them to become more and more knowledgeable, organized, and vocal. Increasingly, they have challenged the traditional authority of medicine (Amara, 1988).

Scandals surrounding medical conduct in research were exposed, further weakening society's faith in organized, institutional medicine (see Jaroff, 1991). The fraud case of Stephen Breuning in 1987 regarding treatment for mentally retarded children has received substantial media attention and provoked bitter debates among medical researchers (Brand, 1987; Roman, 1988; Valentine, 1988). The charges against Robert Gallo regarding the alleged scientific misconduct of his research team in the discovery of HIV have also appeared (Crewdson, 1989; Roberts, 1990). In addition, concern has escalated that medical researchers' financial links to large industries may lead them, for economic and not medical reasons, to distort scientific findings in order to bolster publicity and the alleged benefits of certain drugs over others. One example is Genentech, Inc.'s drug TPA for treating heart diseases. It was revealed that a majority of principal investigators of the drug at the National Institutes of Health owned stock in the biotech company. A powerful financial incentive thus existed for them to pursue the marketing approval of the drug aggressively (Carey, 1990, p. 148). U.S. Representative John D. Dingell commented on these scandals: "The highest value in science should be truth, but we have examined cases which indicate that scientists may be more concerned with money, self-preservation, and obfuscation" (quoted in Carey, 1990, p. 145).

Sociological and critical analyses of medicine have offered a range of models challenging medicine's historical position of authority. For instance, the notion of "discovery" in biomedicine has been profoundly problematized (Reines, 1991). A whole literature has long existed that argues for the model of "accidental discovery" in science, thereby challenging researchers' claims of control, rationality, even authenticity (Cannon, 1945; Comroe, 1977; Dale, 1948). The problem of medical discovery has also been interpreted by scholars as a socially constructed process, using narrative theory (Myers, 1990; Nash, 1990), psycholinguistic theory (Nickles, 1985), socioecological theory (Lederberg, 1988; Price, 1989), and so on.

The most disturbing criticism of medical science regards its inability to deliver care. As Fox (1988) has argued, "Medical scientists proved to be better at basic research and at devising new technologies for diagnosis and for keeping very sick patients alive than at finding cures" (p. 322).

Similarly, Lewis Thomas argues that most of what is propagated as "high science" in medicine is mostly a set of technological equipments for diagnostic precision. He maintains that these "many exquisite refinements of our methods for detecting biochemical abnormalities of one sort or another . . . have not yet been matched by any comparable transformations in therapy" (1988, p. 385). These technologies are used "to shore up things after the still-unexplained diseases of these organs have run their course" (p. 386). Moreover, these measures account for a large portion of the ever-rising costs of health care today. In light of these ongoing crises in public health and biomedicine, the Clinton administration's public health reform efforts (still in the making at this writing) are the most visible attempt in recent years to salvage the public's faith in the authority of medicine as a whole.

To consider medicine's response to the AIDS crisis, we must turn to this much wider terrain of historical forces I have roughly sketched here. We must turn away, momentarily, from the question of how medicine responds to AIDS specifically, to how it responds to a deeper crisis (one that precedes AIDS) via its response to this immediate crisis. I am suggesting that the AIDS crisis emerges, not from nowhere, but out of an already widespread crisis of the social and political authority of medicine. The crisis is now constructed to link up, not to nowhere, but to the stable definitions of curability/incurability, which present the historical possibility of managing the authority of medicine. As a result, medicine seeks to manage not only the present crisis of AIDS but also that other, deeper crisis of authority, through the problematic "reform" of the clinical trials method, the attempt to delegitimize alternative theories and treatment methods, and, as we shall see in this chapter, the counterchallenge to the AIDS treatment activist movement.

To be perfectly clear, I am arguing that the so-called AIDS crisis was in part *produced* as a focal point for the attempt to relegitimize organized, institutional, and technological medicine in a society that had grown skeptical of it prior to AIDS. All of this is part of the discourse of curing AIDS. All of it requires an explanation and analysis beyond the specific struggles of AIDS treatment. All of it suggests that the pair of contradictory discourses of AIDS has something to do with the crises and management of hegemony.

The question is whether this hegemonic struggle for authority means that the social and medical policies developed in the search for AIDS treatment have now been complicated by other structural motives and interests of power. Most important, we must consider whether these issues of power are enabling or impeding the urgent task of developing effective therapeutic treatment for AIDS. The plethora of problems in AIDS treatment research—including the usual delay of testing and approval of drugs, the incredible fluctuation of funding for AIDS research, and the failure of the FDA and the NIH to respond to the requests of PWAs—may indeed be the result of a medical system struggling to resuscitate its authority at this historical conjuncture. In this way, despite technomedicine's drastic failure to produce a "cure" or to alleviate the burdens of health care significantly, it continues to see AIDS as an opportunity—indeed, a prime target—for reversing its ailing authority.

## Between Technomedicine and AIDS Treatment Activism

By now it is impossible to think of technomedical authority without considering its relationship to the gay male subject. It has been made clear that the way gay men and AIDS have been unambiguously connected from the outset has less to do with homosexuality than with how it is constellated in the (homophobic) conditions of our culture (despite the suggestion by physicians and journalists that certain gay sexual activities may have been linked to the disease). Does the "fact" of curing AIDS, too, arise from a field of meaning connotatively loaded with reference to homosexuality? Can the question of how technomedicine responds to AIDS be separated from the question of how medicine—as a social institution as well as a political entity allied with powerful socioeconomic groups—views homosexuality? Is "curing AIDS" being meshed with "curing/controlling" homosexuality, given that both have been historically situated in the domain of "medical research"? Could we argue that this connection provides an element of psychosocial homogeneity necessary for the relegitimation of medical authority? Given that medicine has had the authority to define, monitor, and control issues of health, and given that it has largely regarded homosexuality as a pathological deviation from health (see Schwanberg, 1990), the whole question of treatment in the AIDS crisis is tainted with electrifying political implications.

In raising these questions, I am strongly suggesting a hypothesis that the biomedical responses to AIDS, however fractured and uneven, have continuously excited an imagination of a repathologization of homosexuality. Again and again we have witnessed a backlash not against the gay communities as such, but against the political position of the AIDS treatment activist movement. The way it is constructed in the dominant media and discussed among medical circles reflects a growing sentiment that treatment activism—usually identified as no different from the "gay movement"—may be threatening the proper conduct of science and jeopardizing the goodwill of medicine. What is jeopardizing good science, it then appears, is the activist movement, and by implication, its underlying "gay agenda."

"ACT UP is merely the latest chapter in the political mobilization of the gay community," writes a reporter (Crossen, 1989). In the news, AIDS activism is grossly conflated with a "gay movement" that is rarely defined, despite the feverish debates among activists to separate the agenda of AIDS-specific activism from that of the general gay-rights activism. This self-conscious separation is often carried out in debates that fracture the activist groups themselves.[1] "Gay rage" has become the common signifier for gay political activism and AIDS activism, now codified in a unification through sickness, desperation, even violence.[2]

After more than seven years of AIDS activism, the dominant media still consistently ignore the enormously positive contributions to the drug development process brought about by the energetic and multifronted actions of the AIDS treatment activists. The press coverage of ACT UP often constructs it as a "special interest" group whose rising political power, which is always coded as civil disobedience, must be closely guarded, as if saying, "Watch out! Here come the radicals!"[3] A member of the studio audience in a *Phil Donahue Show* that featured a panel of ACT UP members (February 9, 1990) shouted: "Stock exchanges and cathedrals—where do you stop? Bombs, buildings? Militancy can turn into terrorism." It has been suggested that the rise of ACT UP's power is inextricably linked with a subversive and violent gay agenda (Kupelian et al., 1990). Negative descriptions of ACT UP abound, and many invoke images of the terrorist, the anarchist, the pervert, or the primitive warrior:

- "A politically savvy group of sick people"; "a gangster group"; "The Revolt of the Ill"; "the gay community's shock troops in the war against AIDS"
- Protest as "guerrilla theater"; "ritual dance, composed with whistles, drums, chanting"; "made-for-TV troublemaking"; "a mixture of the shrill and the shrewd"; "hate rally"; protest doubles as "a pro-sex campaign"

- Actions as "militant eroticism"; actions "trespass the bounds of good taste"; actions as "outlet for its members' anger and fear about dying at an early age"
- Tactics were "sexually explicit"; "irresponsible and inappropriate"; "unconventional and irreverent"
- Confrontation as "poisonous phone calls and face-to-face abuse"
- Regular meetings "bristle with conspiracy theories and paranoia"; regular meetings as "an exercise in creative anarchy"
- Protest site as "zoo" or "madhouse of the 'AIDS gulag' "
- "Most of [ACT UP's] power comes from menace"
- Activists "confuse" political action with "cathartic psychotherapy"
- "State-of-the-art media manipulation"
- "Virtually impossible to please" [4]

A sample of newspaper headlines reveals similarly ghoulish descriptions:

"AIDS Guerrillas" (*New York*, November 12, 1990)

"ACT UP Acts Out: Crossing the 'Revulsion Threshold' " (*Commonweal*, September 14, 1990)

"When Activism Becomes Gangsterism" (*U.S. News & World Report*, February 5, 1990)

"Acting Up to Fight AIDS: A Group's Angry Tactics" (*Newsweek*, June 6, 1988)

"Uncivil Disobedience: This AIDS Extremist is for Riots and Assassination" (*Mother Jones*, November-December 1990)

"Shock Troops: AIDS Activist Group Harasses and Provokes to Make Its Point" (*Wall Street Journal*, December 7, 1989)

"Rude, Rash, Effective, ACT UP Shifts AIDS Policy" (*New York Times*, January 3, 1990)

More structured commentaries about ACT UP in a set of antitheses that divide the activists along arbitrary lines are as follows:

1. *Active/Passive.* A major way in which AIDS activism is signified as eroding the symbolic threshold of social tolerance is the distinction between its various forms of protest. Generally, silent peaceful marches are preferred to active interventions. A reporter reflects on the Sixth International Conference on AIDS in San Francisco, June 1990:

No longer are AIDS protesters content with poignant candlelight marches to mourn the dead or quiet negotiation with public health officials. Now they breach barricades near the doors at the opening ceremonies here, occupy the hotel that is conference headquarters until organizers agree to more free passes, disrupt delegates' cocktail parties and stage rude street theater and acts of civil disobedience that dominate the evening news. (Gross, 1990a)

News photographs make this distinction as well. Frequently, images of protesters as angry, radical-looking, finger-pointing hooligans are juxtaposed with pictures of subdued gay men hugging one another or kneeling in sorrow, usually before the backdrop of the Names Project Quilt display. Captions also signify the difference; for example, "Trespassing the bounds of good taste: New York protest" (Salholz et al., 1988) against "A decade of death: Mourners at the AIDS quilt in Washington" (Salholz et al., 1990).

2. *Inside/Outside.* This specific spatial marking delineates the symbolic boundary of society's tolerance of the activists' actions. Commentators have objected that protests frequently intrude into spaces sanctioned for "civil" gathering. In effect, they suggest that street protests are more tolerated than "invasive" protests. The response to ACT UP's demonstration in St. Patrick's Cathedral on December 10, 1989, typifies this opinion (DeParle, 1990; Leo, 1990). Another audience member in the February 9, 1990, ACT UP episode of the *Phil Donahue Show* mentioned earlier in this chapter argued that moving inside the church was perceived as the equivalent of defaming the church. Taking up the liberal consultant's role, he advised: "I think their action is wrong. Stay outside the church, be very vocal, get out there with pamphlets." Similar responses were expressed toward ACT UP's protests at conference sites (Barinaga, 1990; Shilts, 1989b).

3. *Separationists/Assimilationists.* This is perhaps the most politically divisive distinction. It constructs lines of allegiance along the sharpest points of difference that activists themselves tend to fight over (the controversy over outing is the obvious example). In delineating the difference between those who believe in practicing their "subversive strategies" and "alternative life-style" from those who choose to restrain from them, the media has constructed gay identity with the "subcultural model" and the "respectable gay model." The former echoes the discourse of promiscuity that embodies a militant-erotic excess. The latter seeks to rehabilitate the ideal of monogamy; it is a redemptive path offered by the mainstream heterosexual life-style, often de-eroticized, domesticated, and most of all signified as a "safe" life-style.

For example, a special issue of *Newsweek* entitled "The Future of Gay America" opens with a discussion of AIDS activism and quickly moves into a discussion of the transformation of gays as a result of the AIDS crisis. It argues that a "gayby boom" has occurred; there is now a new generation of gays who are discreet, coupled, monogamous, cohabitating, career-oriented, and interested in family and domestic affairs. It describes them as participating in "marriage hetero style" and "living the settled-down life of their 'breeder' peers" (Salholz et al., 1990, p. 25). The report is accompanied by two sets of photographs. The first includes an image of a group of protesting activists shot in a wide lens, exaggerating their protruding bodies and postures, and an image of two gay men in a dimly lit bar, caressing each other, both drinking. The second set includes a picture of a lesbian couple picnicking in a park and feeding their adopted child, and a picture of a gay male couple also with their adopted children, shot in the classic "family portrait" style. We are thus offered polarized prototypes of gay people, one to be exalted for its emulation of the heterosexual models, the other to be rejected for its moral bankruptcy.

All of the antitheses discussed here are those frequently taken up in the debates within gay communities and among ACT UP members. Yet the mainstream press has already constructed what is considered proper and what is not: those who choose to be "outside," "passive," and "assimilationist" tend to be more "socially tolerable." The preferred images of gays offer a social spectacle of a "cured" homosexuality. A "healthy lifestyle" now has a double meaning.

Inversely, the image of the "homosexual activists" signifies degeneracy and general unhealthiness. The most politically repellent construction of AIDS activists is found in the extremist magazine *New Dimension*. The magazine, originating in Oregon, has published numerous issues devoted entirely to AIDS. In the wake of Oregon's draconianly homophobic legislature, the readership of the magazine is increasing. *New Dimension*'s essays use misinformation and false accusations to decry that "homosexual activists" are gaining power and skewing public health policies in selfish directions, thereby undermining scientific integrity.

> While the ascension of gays to positions of power in the AIDS establishment started off as a seemingly positive development in the fight against AIDS, over time a bizarre recurring pattern has emerged. Incredible as it seems, by almost all accounts, *priority one* for the militant gay AIDS activists is *not* so much the preservation of life, even their own, through

adhering to proven public health measures, but rather, the preservation and promotion of the homosexual lifestyle itself—at all costs. (Kupelian et al., 1990, p. 23; emphasis in the original)

Similarly offensive rhetoric in the same issue compares AIDS activists with "nagging children":

> On the socio-political level, if the members of any social order give in to the little provocations of subversive political factions, sooner or later they will collectively surrender their emotional energies and finances to the spoiled "militant special interest groups." For these groups, enough is never enough, and . . . society has learned to cope with the unrelenting intimidation of these self-centered pressure groups by denying that there could be anything wrong with these groups. (Masters, 1990, p. 45)

A political backlash against the image and political position of the gay communities is being launched, based on the construction that they threaten a "proper" scientific control of the epidemic and that they propagate a "gay agenda" beneath the facade of the treatment activism movement. The wolf is hiding underneath the sheepskin. An old tale indeed.

The systematic attack of the AIDS activist movement is strongest on the point of treatment issues. The attack is usually mounted upon three objections. First, it is felt that AIDS activists threaten the scientific standard of drug approval. The activists' effort to transform the medical establishment is often misdescribed as an effort to overthrow it entirely (Thompson, 1990a). Second, it has been argued that AIDS activists tend to overstate the scope of the epidemic. Funding for AIDS is often compared with funding for other diseases in order to suggest that AIDS has somehow robbed from other diseases. In contrasting AIDS with heart disease (the most common comparison), Michael Fumento, author of *The Myth of Heterosexual AIDS*, argues: "It is wrong to spend more money on a disease [AIDS] that will never kill more than 35,000 to 40,000 people a year than on a disease [heart disease] that will kill a half-million every year" (cited in Thompson, 1990a, p. 24). This comment typifies a model now generally adopted by the AIDS medical establishment that takes the death toll as an index of what needs to be done and how much funding a disease should receive. It refuses to use the number of lives saved as a basis for making those judgments. It also ignores that genetic and immunological research spawned by AIDS can and does often benefit research concerning other diseases (see Carpenter, 1989; Jaroff, 1990; Murphy, 1991). Biomedical research cannot be narrowly compartmentalized. Ironically, the accusation that AIDS research is over-funded reveals it as one of the only areas of biomedical research that approaches having adequate funding ("Dying for Dollars," 1990). In this regard, the attack on AIDS activists as struggling for funding for AIDS at the expense of ignoring other diseases is absurd.

The third and perhaps the strongest accusation against AIDS activists regarding treatment is that they have distorted the "proper" public health response to the crisis by shifting attention away from prevention to treatment effort.

> No one can deny that AIDS victims deserve all the compassion and help that society can muster. . . . But . . . the focus on present suffering may be diverting too much attention from the task of protecting those who could become victims. . . . Prevention is vital because a cure is still distant, if it is attainable at all. (Thompson, 1990b, pp. 42-43)

Society still cannot conceive of prevention and treatment together. The separation of "general" and "special" interests remains one of the deep-est barriers for a coordinated public health system. The scientists' and journalists' accusations that AIDS activists are close minded and irre-sponsible are painfully ironic when a government and a medical estab-lishment still refuse to provide equitable health care and are still inca-pable of breaking down fundamental prejudices against gays and other minority groups struck by AIDS. The accusations also ignore the enor-mous progress made by activists' broad-based and well-educated inter-vention in prevention *and* treatment.

In the attack on the AIDS treatment activist movement, we witness not only an endemic demonization of the movement but the violence of a society directed at people who, having been savagely hated and brutally shunned away, are not regarded as worthy of living and fighting back. At the heart of this violence, we confront political realities that have emerged around the new historical shifts of gay subjectivity.

## "Curing" AIDS and "Postmodern" Gay Subjectivities

In the conjunctural moments when, on the one hand, technomedicine is "reproducing" AIDS as the focal point in its struggle over its own crisis of authority, and, on the other hand, AIDS activism is generally attacked for its subversion of the authority of technomedicine, the imagination of a unified "gay subject" must be, and in fact has been, effectively dismantled. To the degree that the AIDS crisis has identified gay men as its prime subject, a vast array of possible social identities is now made possible, or has been constructed, for them. A consideration of the question of gay subjectivity can further illuminate the conjunctural nature of the discourse of "curing" AIDS, for the very notion of gay subjectivity is at the moment in the making.

At one level, the terms of curability/incurability have cast gays as both the subjects of morbid death and devastation and the objects of scientific and health education inquiries. The mobilization of the lethal fantasy of massive gay death, if not extinction, is in fact remarkably consistent with the logic of containment. By constituting gays as scientific objects whose "scientific value" lies more in their imminent death (the disappearing subjects in clinical drug trials) than in their chance of survival, and as examples of self-destruction, remorse, and repentance in health education, the logic of containment constructs gays (particularly gay men) as subjects outside the symbolic realm of "curing." Especially in the early years of the epidemic, gay men appeared at scientific conferences and public health education forums only as the augurers of the grave, their bodies—more specifically, the synecdochal form of anal intercourse—the sign of the incurable.

At another level, however, the shifting conjunction between technomedicine and AIDS treatment activism has found gay men in less easily definable positions. If my suggestion that technomedicine is currently involved in a hegemonic struggle for its own authority is accurate, then I further suggest that in this emerging hegemonic field is an attempt to resurrect the gay subject as part of the technocratic force. The social demonizing of the figure of the gay AIDS activist has opened a space for the construction of a more socially "tolerable" and more "gentle" figure of the gay activist, who, by virtue of being a survivor in the crisis (but still a dying subject) can emerge as a useful ally, even as a "partner" in the technocratic structure responsible for developing AIDS treatment. The courting of gay activists by the scientific establishment—as guest panelists at scientific conferences, consultants on task forces, or liaisons to the PWA communities—coincides with the gay activists' own attempt to professionalize themselves so as to gain legitimacy in the scientific discourse of AIDS. In both instances, the apparent erosion of the political division between technomedicine and AIDS activism, the result not only of a strategic reterritorialization by the scientific establishment but also of the heroic vigilance of the activists in breaking down the stereotype of

PWAs as victims, has shaped a postmodern gay subject who possesses a relative degree of fluidity in moving across various social and symbolic spaces. This postmodern gay subject, by virtue of being a relational subject, cannot override the transcendental fantasies of morbidity/containment, even as it reshapes the effect of these fantasy structures. That is, it arises not from any possible path of imagination (as the term postmodern may suggest) but from the vantage point of the fantasy scenes that find the tropes of gay death, gay genocide, gay as scientific object, and the self-redemptive gay as its representations.

In the inauguration of the "new" gay subject in the conjunctural moment of hegemony, gay men continue to find that our highly ambivalent relations and feelings to technomedicine, to health education efforts, to scientific journalism, and even to the oppressive figure of morbidity have in the course of the crisis been magnified. Our feelings are ambivalent because we have not forgotten—indeed, we have been constantly reminded of—the uneasy position of an entire historical constituency secured (in both the sense of being fastened or trapped and being offered a space in discourse) in the hands of physicians, scientists, bureaucrats, and journalists. As the hegemonic project of technomedicine proceeds, the emblem of "Silence = Death," critically central to (but not limited to) the political articulation of gay activism, seems to have reappeared as a figure of ambivalence. As the activists have constructed a subject position that negates silence to counteract death—that is, a subject position that validates discourse to affirm life—they have gradually realized that discourse itself incites many different lives, not all of which confirm an activist pose, not all of which result in an oppositional politic in its traditional sense. Larry Kramer, for instance, has over the years continued to break the figure of silence in order to enact an activist discourse that has at its center not the figure of life, but the figure of guilt associated with self-inflicted death among gays as a rhetorical motor for his vision of AIDS activism. His persistent words "We're killing each other. Can't you see that?" addressed to gay men are never directed at the "life-style issues" assumed to be connected to the risks of death. Nor, in more recent occasions, are they even directed at gay men's complacency and apathy assumed (by Kramer) to be a sure cause of defeat and demise. Rather, Kramer's activist discourse is specifically directed at the fraction of the AIDS activist movement assumed by him to have relinquished its oppositional power by making alliances with the mainstream technocratic force. In Kramer's discourse, what counts as a gay male subject—

assuming an uncomplicated reality of being a survivor in the crisis—is the militant oppositional political subject.

Another activist, Douglas Crimp, argues that the reinvention of the gay male subject in the conjuncture of the AIDS crisis need not be essentialized to the militant subject position. He challenges the assumption that "silence" in "Silence = Death" permanently signifies an antiactivist quietism: "We ourselves are silent precisely on the subject of death, on how deeply it affects us" (Crimp, 1989, p. 4). Crimp sees a "silent subject" as important in the complex reality of AIDS activism against the savage assault on gay men and on the entire gay culture; in his view, many gay men find even survival in the crisis—the fact of having a subjectivity, of being a subject alive amid death—an ambivalent status to bear. He asks provocatively, "But how are we to dissociate our narcissistic satisfaction in being alive from our fight to stay alive? And, insofar as we *identify* with those who have died, how can our satisfactions in being alive escape guilt at having survived?" (p. 9). In the discourse, such as Kramer's, that adamantly rejects a nonmilitant, nonoppositional subject position lies a miscalculation of the magnitude of psychosocial ambivalence experienced by gay men. For those "paralyzed with fear, filled with remorse, or overcome with guilt" (p. 16)—psychic responses resulting from gay men's collective subject position enacted around "mourning"— the militant subject position may be unaccommodating, if not unimaginable. Crimp's plea for "militancy, of course, then, but mourning too: mourning *and* militancy" (p. 18) opens an important path for thinking about the need, sometimes, to occupy a tacitly politicized subject position essential to our overall struggle to cope with the crisis. A bifurcated subject position of mourning/militancy can be considered part of the postmodern gay male subject. It would not at all be surprising that in the gay communities' reinvention of their relations to technomedicine, health education, and the media, the figures of the ally, the professional, and the partner coexist with those of the mourner and the militant activist not in a sense of mutuality or even schizophrenia, but in a strategic appropriation couched in the communities' own forms of moralism, pathos, and faith. All of this suggests that even within the powerfully lethal hold of the fantasy of gay death (which can be traced in both Kramer's and Crimp's versions of gay activism), we do not always know in advance the multiple effects of the lines that divide cooperation from opposition, silence from discourse, passivity from activism.

Such an ambivalence has been constellated and reconstellated in the "gay moment" apparently excited by the politics of the Clinton administration (see Kopkind, 1993). The embrace of such a cultural and political moment for gay people, however, has appeared amid skepticism, because, once again, we cannot predict the political effects of the "mainstreaming" or "normalizing" of homosexuality. Clinton's interest in such a mainstreaming or normalization of gays (however unenthusiastic at times) appears simultaneously with his health care reform agenda. The flurry of debates around health care reform in early 1993, at the time of this writing, seemed to make visible the hegemonic struggle by technomedicine to regain authority in an ambivalent climate of long-term frustration and distrust, and renewed faith and hope. President Clinton's attempt to feature health care reform as a major political agenda in his early days in office strongly suggested the ascension of a remedicalized polity that apparently finds in the relegitimation of an ailing technomedical institution (its technocratic professionalism, its ability to incite the figure of the medical subject, even as a political subject, and its general ability to reconfigure an ailing economy) a golden opportunity to reinvent a "democratic" culture.

Like most White House politics, however, Clinton's failure to see the interconnection of the proposal for health care reform and the proposal to transform gay civil rights (and the civil rights of women and other oppressed constituencies) reflects his pathetically weak leadership in fighting AIDS. As prominently as the discourses of gay rights and medical reform feature in mainstream political discussions today, the appalling lack of a comprehensive AIDS agenda from the Clinton administration not only points to a betrayal of the gay constituencies, who extended major support to the Clinton/Gore ticket, and to the lethal reality of conservative pressures persistently attempting to mold a centrist political platform for the administration but suggests that in the liberal struggle for a "democratic" politics and culture, the gay constituencies still do not feature—indeed, are not yet allowed to feature—as a central subject in the reform of technomedical and other issues. To the degree that gay activists have over the years successfully articulated a feasible democratic discourse for AIDS, particularly for the problem of AIDS treatment, their voice is rendered fragile around the highly ambivalent status of the postmodern gay subject.

The artifact that is the "postmodern gay subject," which can stage a political assault to the mad fantasy of an erasure of gay subject altogether in the virulent discourses of morbidity/containment, may by the same positioning reify these master discourses that reinstall the gay subject as a major link in the conjunctural hegemonic crisis over the reestablishment of a hypermedicalized democratic culture.

# 5 An Epistemology of Curing

The only theory worth having is that which you have to fight off, not
that which you speak with profound fluency.
Stuart Hall, "Cultural Studies and Its Theoretical Legacies"

Perhaps our hopes for accountability for techno-biopolitics in the belly
of the monster turn on revisioning the world as coding trickster with
whom we must learn to converse.
Donna Haraway, "The Promises of Monsters"

Like a catfish, I feed off others' castoffs; I am less interested in cultural
forms as something *for me* to interpret than I am in listening as other
people offer their interpretations of them. . . . River bottom-feeding, I
swallow [the cultural forms'] meanings and try to figure out what sort of
sense they make.
Jan Zita Grover, "AIDS, Keywords, and Cultural Work"

Staring at the monitor of my computer, caught in sentimental ambivalence embodied in the scratchy voice and soul of Tina Turner as she sings,
"What's love got to do with it?" on my CD player nearby, I ask a similarly sentimental and ambivalent question: What's theory got to do with
it? As I have attempted in this book to track, report, interpret, and analyze the languages and practices associated with the phenomenon of
"curing" AIDS as (and after) they erupt into our public and private consciousness, I undertake this project as someone who, in large part, watches other people swim. These people (and the metaphor of swimming)
come vividly alive in Jan Zita Grover's (1992) admirable essay "AIDS,
Keywords, and Cultural Work" as images of the physicians who develop
new ways of treating opportunistic infections, the hospital staff members
who are less reluctant now to perform their duties in the AIDS wards of
their hospital, or the volunteers and activists who are getting burned out;
as abstract images of "ordinary" people "who work in conventional jobs
in business and government [and] go home afterward and choose to do
the brainwork in the evenings and weekends"; and, finally, as the image
of Grover herself as a volunteer in AIDS agencies, an editor of a community newspaper, and a cultural critic. To the degree that these are images
of workers and work located, in a manner of speaking, in the trenches of
the AIDS war zone—reflections in the swimming pool—the crisis known

as "AIDS" begs the question not of "what" but of "*how* has theory got to do with it?" And because the crisis is complex and multifronted, no one way can best assess the usefulness of theory. Let me add here that I (and I suspect a few other academically oriented writers like me) am afraid of swimming, and, to a lesser extent, of the water itself. I contend that, as much as we need a way to describe, however nervously, the psychic economy of AIDS for the various communities affected by it, we also need a way to describe it for those who are afraid.

In this final chapter, I take as a self-evident premise that "technomedicine is a discursive practice" and as a bold assumption that "AIDS is culture." Rooted, at least for now, in this premise and assumption, this chapter will attempt to retrace the theoretical trajectory that has framed this book. The first of the two sections of this chapter will offer a brief and fairly straightforward summary of some of the cultural criticisms that have emerged around AIDS so as to identify the major theoretical propositions and problematics presented in these works. I will limit my discussion to the theoretical works that take the representation of the crisis by the mass media (particularly the news) as their object of criticism. This brief excursion will help to clarify the more specific theoretical territory I would like to locate this book, via Michel Foucault's theory of discourse and the theory of articulation of British cultural studies.

The second section will sketch some theoretical axioms about the concept of "curing." Some of these axioms are recapitulations of the theoretical notions already scattered throughout this book; others will provide additional and related perspectives to help us understand the problem of "curing" a bit more clearly. These axioms will contribute to the overall heterogeneous and lively debates surrounding AIDS as a whole, particularly those akin to "cultural studies." Of course, I realize that these undertakings occur only in the belly of the monster.

### Critical Analyses of the Media Representations of AIDS: An Overview

By now, it is a common recognition that the media have done a remarkably poor job of reporting AIDS, especially during the early years of the epidemic. Many media research studies have drawn this conclusion, finding the media's coverage flawed by sensationalism, melodrama, stigmatization, and inaccuracy. Many recent works have analyzed AIDS in the media by using traditional frameworks of mass communication research, including agenda-setting theory (Colby and Cook, 1991, 1992; Dearing

and Rogers, 1988); social problems theory (Baker, 1986); political communication (Altman, 1986; Buxton, 1991; Juhasz, 1992; Lerner, 1991;
McAllister, 1990); and content analysis (Albert, 1986a, 1986b; Goldstein, 1991; Karpf, 1988; Kinsella, 1989; Saalfield, 1990; Saalfield and
Navarro, 1991; Schwartz, 1984). Some have combined mass communication theory with discourse theory (Patton, 1990). The empirical findings of these studies can provide us with a concrete map of how AIDS
became public knowledge through the media. They also reveal some of
the irreversible damage done to the social perception of AIDS and people
with AIDS. Although I have referred to some of this information in earlier chapters, I think a brief summary will prove useful:

1. The language of reporting tended to be euphemistic ("the exchange
of bodily fluids"), mystifying ("guilty victims," "general population"),
and inaccurate (the "AIDS test," the "AIDS virus," "HIV virus").

2. Reporting tended to be reactive rather than proactive. Short-lived
and often decontextualized reporting triggered by specific and highly
"newsworthy" events (such as the story of Rock Hudson, or blood con-
tamination stories) was plentiful compared to in-depth and analytical
reporting (for example, Crewdson, 1989).

3. Reporting latched onto and perpetuated a rigid social hierarchy,
always coded in binary terms: innocent/guilty, heterosexual/homosexu-
al, exposed/closet, First World/Third World.

4. Reporting was cyclical because the media felt compelled to regulate itself so as to avoid creating panic in the public.

5. AIDS has been conventionally linked with homosexuality in the
media.

6. Because of the link of AIDS with homosexuality, the media virtually ignored the crisis until research showed that the population outside of
the gay communities could contract the disease.

7. Promiscuity was often the dominant focus in the discussion of
homosexuality, purportedly the sociological index of a repulsive,
deviant life-style.

8. The image of gays infected with the virus was consistently cast in a
negative light: they were "burned out" by their own fast-lane life-style;
they were abandoned by their friends and families; they were terrorized
and devastated by their own sickness; some continued to engage in
"dangerous" sex; others regretted and denounced their former life-style.

All of these depictions contributed to the repathologization of homosexuality.

9. AIDS activism has often been confused with gay activism.

10. The visibility of AIDS/gay activisms was said to produce contradictory effects: it further linked homosexuality with AIDS, yet it also raised public awareness and stimulated scientific interests in developing treatments for the disease.

11. Human-interest stories, which have multiplied since the breaking of the Rock Hudson story, tended to adopt an interrogative mode focused less on reporting the experience of the illness of PWAs than on generating confession, remorse, and regret of their "life-style" before their illness. The "real" interest, it seemed, was to present PWAs as pitiful objects for the general public's "compassionate" look.

12. Firmly fixed in the future tense, the press always turned to rhetorical constructs such as projections, statistical speculations, and the construction of doomsday scenarios.

13. Journalists depended heavily on medical authorities to shape and control reporting. A small group of "experts" emerged as regularly featured spokespersons. The dependence on medical sources contributed to the phenomenon of medicalization, whereby the disease was accented with moral/medical implications.[1]

As these findings indicate, the media's news programs seem to have offered the same conventional, simplified, and formulaic ideas about AIDS, particularly during the early years of the epidemic. Paula Treichler succinctly characterizes the coverage:

> Patterns of AIDS coverage on the networks are at times so identical that one imagines their representatives all at the same AIDS workshop—learning how to give events the same conventional interpretations, select the same AIDS experts, use the same misleading terminology, and track down the same live footage from the people who were *really* there. (1989a, p. 147)

The stigmatization and sensationalism reveal not so much intentionality or prejudice among journalists (although these exist too) as the shifting constellation of forces that dominate, shape, and mobilize the often culturally and politically negative responses to AIDS. The pitiful record of the media coverage of AIDS in fact raises concerns about the relations between language, power, and the body; in short, about the cultural politics of representation.

The question of representation has been a central preoccupation of the growing body of cultural criticisms focusing on AIDS, whose basis is the realization that representation, and language in general, is a place where the possibility for struggle can be realized. If AIDS has indeed emerged as a focal point for the political control of identity and subjectivity and the repression of the body and desire—and the media's systematically biased and sensationalized coverage of AIDS provides ample evidence to support this point—then we must politicize representation. We must theorize how representation works as well as how oppositional politics can be mounted against the consistently demeaning and disempowering representations of AIDS. Treichler has argued that we cannot look through representation to discover what AIDS "really" means. Instead, we must turn to representation itself as the very site where such a discovery can take place (1988, p. 195). In other words, representation is the very point where we can determine reality, the most powerful tool with which we can conceptualize the meaning and the social effects of AIDS. More important, given that the material power to alter the conditions of the crisis is consistently denied to many of us affected by the crisis, representation provides a crucial space for intervention and contestation. Video activist Stuart Marshall argues that this space is provided by

> those media—performance, visual arts, video, film, printed media— through which the AIDS-affected communities can and do address themselves. Only through these media is there a possibility of opening up the contradictions within the apparent homogeneity of medical discourse or of producing radically different conceptualizations of the body, disease and health. (1990, p. 36)

The two main strands of critical work appear in an increasing number of essays and in many significant anthologies, among them those edited by Boffin and Gupta (1990), Carter and Watney (1989), Crimp (1987), Fuss (1991), Klusacek and Morrison (1992), Miller (1992), and Murphy and Poirier (1993). The first strand studies the media coverage of AIDS by linking a cultural theory of representation with psychoanalytic theories. This is most evident in the work of AIDS activist and scholar Simon Watney. Watney wants to situate the problem of ideology as it relates to the politics of the representation of gay identities at the level of psychic formations. He argues in the preface to the second edition of *Policing Desire: Pornography, AIDS, and the Media* that he is

firmly convinced of the need to address questions concerning the operations of fantasy and the unconscious in relation to our (provisional)
understanding of the political and ideological economies of this epidemic.
If anything the need for a psychoanalytic perspective is more pressing than
before, given the nature of the belated responses to AIDS from mainstream criticism, sociology, historiography, and so on. (1989, p. ix)

Watney stresses that the phobic responses to AIDS and homosexuality
from the media and the overall silence of the mainstream establishment
reveal many underlying operations of the unconscious. He elaborates a
theory of the media and its relation to the representation of homosexuality in this way:

> The very existence of homosexual desire, let alone gay identities, are only
> admitted to the frame of mass media representations in densely coded
> forms, which protect the "general public" from any threat of potential
> destabilization. This is the context in which we should think about the cri-
> sis of representation with which AIDS threatens the mass media, under-
> stood above all else as *an agency of collective fantasy*. (1987a, p. 42;
> emphasis added)

The psychoanalytic perspective allows us to see that the media do not
"make" homosexuality into a monstrosity; rather, homosexuality is, and
always has been, felt to be "inherently" monstrous, for it is perceived as
a psychic deviation from the entire collective fantasy of "normal sexuality." Watney argues that this explains why the media feels so compelled
to speak on behalf of the interest of the "family," a mythic concept that
embodies the ideological/psychical existence of that normal sexuality.
Throughout *Policing Desire*, he examines the ideological work done by
the media—particularly the tabloid press—through operations such as
"disavowal," "hysteria," "projection," "disidentification," "repression," "fantasy," and so on. He suggests that psychoanalytic theory can
provide a fuller explanation of the media's homophobic response to
AIDS than can the "moral panic theory" (1987a, p. 43).

A great part of the "psychic formation" that gets organized around
diseases involves the separation of identities and bodies between the sick
and the healthy, that imaginary sense of security of the Self articulated
through the fear, suppression, and rejection of the Other. Sander Gilman
(1988) compares the historical iconography of syphilis with modern popular representations of AIDS. He suggests a strikingly similar structural
operation of Self and Otherness by which AIDS patients, like syphilitics,
are located in relation to the society in which they dwell. The politics of

representation therefore lies in the enactment of boundaries, semiotically as well as psychically, even though the boundaries may be fragile. In Gilman's view, the popular media and the arts have engaged in the cultural and psychical work of boundary making in the specific constructions of the AIDS patients as the melancholic, the sociopathic drug users, the (almost always) blacks, and the contaminated female. Once the images of the afflicted, the ill, or the contaminated are marked and located, we may then mark and locate ourselves in the imaginary space of wellness and wholeness.

But signification must confront the shadow it casts: the meaninglessness that it first rejects but that returns whenever and wherever meaning is bestowed. Meaning making, which largely depends on the construction of positive and negative categories, also creates a negative space that threatens to undermine meaning itself. In other words, when viewed together with psychoanalytic theories, the sociological perspective regarding the problems of alienation and discrimination in the epidemic and the semiotic perspective regarding the construction of Self/Other through signification in fact imply the recognition of the Lack in Kristeva's term, or the abject (the nonobject choice).

Judith Williamson's analysis of the figure of HIV and the psychical formation that is organized around it takes Gilman's thesis one step farther to reveal this overdetermined character of AIDS. She argues that the cultural constructions of HIV embody a psychical split so that HIV is at once full of meaning and hauntingly meaningless. Following up on this idea, I have suggested that the meaningfulness of HIV narratives comes from the way the media adopt the languages of the horror, melodrama, and detective genres already so entrenched in popular discourses, so much so that HIV now possesses a personality, an agenda, and even preferences (see chapter 2). Williamson goes on to argue that at a deeper psychical level, however, the horror of HIV, like the horror of death, threatens to break down all significations, so that a negativity exists that destroys the very artifact that is meaning. We thus cannot talk about the semiotic economy of AIDS (the positive/negative axis) without also examining the psychical economy of AIDS (the meaningfulness/meaninglessness axis). This argument has implications for understanding our subjectivity in relation to AIDS:

> While on the one hand, enlisted to the codes of narrative order, the virus becomes a coherent subject, with schedules, targets and even an admirable

lack of prejudice, on the other it threatens the disintegration of precisely that order of narrative closure which keeps our subjectivity in place—and, in its effects on the body itself, seems to produce the very image of dissolution of the subject, the self as cut out from the world and separate from all that is not-self. (Williamson, 1989, p. 78)

Ultimately, the material body has to confront its inevitable demise, as it tries to defend itself from diseases and those who carry them. Ultimately, the imaginary social categories so aggressively defended and shielded off by the media such as the "family" and "normal sexuality" are rendered fragile. By pointing to this paradox of AIDS embodied in the figure of HIV, Williamson provides a model for understanding the politics of representation and its vulnerability, through the integrative perspectives of linguistics, narrative theories, and psychoanalytic theories.

The first strand of critical analysis of AIDS sees representation as the manifestation of a deep level of anxiety regarding illness, the homosexual Other, and even libidinal desire. According to this view, the media embody that collective anxiety, caught up in the continuously shifting play of dialectic forces that threaten to undermine each other. In many ways, the media's power lies in the way it magnifies, transposes, and diffuses anxiety upon all levels of society. Eventually, the fear of AIDS is articulated as the fear of *both* the Other and the Self.

The second strand of analysis examines the question of power as it relates to the processes of knowledge production. Paula Treichler's work is an example of this kind of analysis. She has largely drawn on feminist theories of language and Foucault's discourse theory to investigate the media's overall constructions of AIDS and how they are articulated with the biomedical discourse of AIDS (1987), the discourse of gender and sexuality in AIDS in popular magazines (1988; 1992b), the discourse of AIDS on network television (1989a), the nationalistic discourse produced in the First World about AIDS in the Third World (1989b), and the construction of gay male identities in the context of AIDS in television melodramas (1993).

Treichler's perspective largely assumes that representation has the power to shape our cultural relationship to the disease and therefore has a directly determining effect on its present and future course. But, as we struggle to grasp the multiple meanings and effects of AIDS produced by the media and biomedical discourses, she argues that finally the disease is "neither directly nor fully knowable" (1988, p. 195). This is because behind any characterization of AIDS, be it scientific discourse or tabloid gossip, there is a history, a culturally evolving set of vocabularies, images, and narratives that may not have their origin in the disease but may arise from entrenched and often contradictory cultural worldviews. Such a theory of representation can explain why even hard scientific facts are always already founded upon existing systems of language. There is no guarantee that these systems of language are compatible with one another; conflicting meanings render any attempt to clearly and fully understand AIDS difficult, if not impossible. As a result, Treichler argues that "we can forget the fight for or against a particular truth and instead interrogate the rules at work in a society that distinguish 'true' representations from 'false' ones" (1989a, p. 150).

Treichler proposes that, following Foucault, we must take AIDS and its many discursive manifestations as objects of knowledge/power. This would enable us to turn away from (mystified) empiricism to ask how that empiricism arises from prior structures of knowledge/power. Specifically, she asks a set of useful questions:

How and why is knowledge about AIDS being produced in the way that it is?
Who is contributing to the process of knowledge production? To whom and by whom is this knowledge disseminated?
What are the practical and material consequences of any new interpretation? Who benefits? Who loses?
On what grounds are facts and truth being claimed? (1988, p. 229)

I suggest that we consider two additional questions. First, how does the knowledge of AIDS gain a strong hold on the body and transform it into an object of social and medical control, not so much through ideology or operations of the unconscious but through the formation of the network of material techniques, procedures, strategies, programs of conduct, and practices of discipline? Behind this question lies the assumption that representation constitutes only one part of the materiality of discourse. The "regime of practices," as phrased by Foucault, creates a discursive formation within which power takes its shape and exercises its authority. The term "discourse" then refers to both the processes of the production of knowledge and subjectivity and the systems of practices. The second additional question we need to ask is, beyond the immediate material effects, what are the overall structural or conjunctural consequences of the production of specific discourses of AIDS? That is, how do discourses rearticulate (realign, reconfigure) the broader constellation of social and political forces in our contemporary history that are both a part of and beyond AIDS? We must theorize representation not only as a matter of significatory and disciplinary relations but also as a matter of historical and, in Gramsci's term, "conjunctural" relations. In this book, I have combined the perspectives of Foucauldian discourse theory and the theory of conjuncturalism to explore the question of "curing AIDS."

### Foucault, Discourse, Practices

What procedures, techniques, technical processes, apparatuses, and programmings of behavior and thought produce knowledge and, more important, produce it as knowledge of truth (rational knowledge)? This question captures a significant portion of Foucault's theoretical paradigm. Throughout his work, he dismantles the normative history of ideas and rationality and asks instead how ideas and rationality emerge within the regimes of truth formed by the network of practices, that is, how they emerge within their "conditions of possibility." Knowledge is, in the deepest sense, practice. In *The Birth of the Clinic*, Foucault has taken great pains to demonstrate that modern medicine was based on a conceptual reorganization of the patient's body from a space that previously could only be reached by physicians through imagination and fantasy to a space that could be penetrated, even "liberated," through the "objective" apparatus of the gaze. Once the importance of medical perception was rejuvenated, a scientifically structured discourse about the patients, their bodies, and their identities could at last be established:

> Medical rationality plunges into the marvelous density of perception, offering the grain of things as the first face of truth, with their colors, their spots, their hardness, their adherence. The breadth of the experiment seems to be identified with the domain of the careful gaze, and of an empirical vigilance receptive only to the evidence of visible contents. The eye becomes the depository and source of clarity; it has the power to bring a truth to light that it receives only to the extent that it has brought it to light; as it opens, the eye first opens the truth. (1975, xiii)

The material procedures and techniques on which this new medical perception was based—the "spatial" classification of diseases and pathological symptoms, the alternation of stages of observation, the dissection of corpses, the reorganization of the hospital field, the integration of the science of observation into medical schools, and so on—became the conditions of possibility for a new medical regime of knowledge/truth.

A practice may be organized around ideological contents and may reflect, deepen, or contradict ideological beliefs, but it cannot be hastily collapsed to the ideological. According to Foucault, the rationality of medical knowledge rests in the immaculate penetration of the tools; the organized experiments; the apparatuses of diagnosis, prescription, and supervision: in short, in the "savage observations" with which the practitioners of medicine open up the body of the patients (1975, p. 30). Whatever "objective truth" of the body is delivered by these practices, it is formed by a network of techniques and programs, not by ideology alone (even though it may be supported by ideology). Scientific medicine is considered a discursive formation, in the sense that the effects of structural practices constitute its own historical conditions of possibility and designate it as positive, believable, and "in the true."

In "Questions of Method," Foucault argues that the question of practices enables us to see the enactment of various historical forms of rationality. Ensembles of techniques are linked to larger, more pervasive systems of truth. Discourse is therefore an aggregate of the technologies of practices (how things operate) and the rise of rationality (what cultural and historical effects of dominance the practices engender). Foucault describes practice as having the "effects of jurisdiction" and rationality as having the "effects of verification" (1981, p. 5), which refer to two corresponding aspects of discourse: what is to be performed and what is to be known. Foucault explains his method of studying discourse as follows:

> If I have studied "practices" like those of the sequestration of the insane, or clinical medicine, or the organization of the empirical sciences, or legal punishment, it was in order to study this interplay between a "code" which rules ways of doing things . . . and a production of true discourses which serve to found, justify, and provide reasons and principles for these ways of doing things. . . . Eventalising singular ensembles of practices, so as to make them graspable as different regimes of "jurisdiction" and "verification." That, to put it in exceedingly barbarous terms, is what I would like to do. (1981, pp. 8-9)

Foucault has thus reinserted the whole question of Truth—defined as the association of a multiplicity of practices to various forms of rationality—into historical and structural analysis. More important, Foucault's emphasis on the question of truth also enables him to theorize power:

> There can be no possible exercise of power without a certain economy of discourses of truth which operates through and on the basis of this association. We are subjected to the production of truth through power and we

cannot exercise power except through the production of truth. . . . In the end, we are judged, condemned, classified, determined in our undertakings, destined to a certain mode of living and dying, as a function of the true discourses which are the bearers of the specific effects of power. (1980, pp. 93-94)

In order to understand Foucault's assertion that power does not take the sole forms of prohibition and repression, we must turn to his theory of truth/rationality to ascertain how truth emerges from the underlying mechanisms and practices that support it.

To return to medical discourse, the central subject of this book, we may now properly situate it in Foucault's theory of discourse. The medical practices and apparatuses that emerged in eighteenth-century France (analyzed in *The Birth of the Clinic*), organized around the structural act of the penetrating gaze on the patient's body, sound familiar as we examine modern technomedicine. AIDS, a disease syndrome whose (supposed) locus of infectivity is a viral agency, a microorganism hidden beneath the immediately graspable surface of the organic body, has quickly rejuvenated medicine's gaze. In medical reports and in the popular media, there is no shortage of (photo)graphic portrayals of the virus buried in the enormous, often black-and-blue-colored space of the inner body. The proliferation of the representations of the virus demonstrates not only the centrality of technovision in modern medicine as a cultural and political practice—the obsession of the gaze, the enactment of scientific rationality over and around the pathological body, the firming-up of the necessity of orthodox science as the preferred response to the crisis—but the representations are also often the pretext for actualizing a set of technical and empirical procedures, rules, and programs used to develop AIDS treatment. We have seen the cultural representations of HIV as they form the ground, the empirical evidence, for producing a regime of practices around "curing" (chapter 2), which dominates a clinicoempirical discourse embodied in the practices of the clinical trial further elaborated in chapter 3.

### Toward a Conjunctural Theory of Frontier Politics

Discourses create and re-create worlds. An underlying assumption of this book is that the cultural notions and practices specific to AIDS always exceed the disease itself. Like pebbles dropped in a pool, the cacophonic images and narratives of AIDS and the complex practices around AIDS reverberate into larger historical themes, potentially realigning the constellation of historical forces already implicated in the crisis. Rooted in this assumption, I suggest that the theory of articulation, as developed by Stuart Hall and others associated with British cultural studies, can help us account for the dynamic historicization of discourse.

The theory of articulation was offered as a result of Hall's rereading of the two central paradigms that characterized cultural studies: culturalism and (post)structuralism. This is evident in his reassessment of Williams's humanism, Althusser's structural Marxism, and poststructuralist discourse theory (of, for instance, Foucault, Laclau, and Derrida) through the work of Gramsci. Hall pays attention to the concrete "strategies" of articulation, among them the specific mechanisms by which articulation operates in the media. A detailed discussion of these strategies and mechanisms appears in *Policing the Crisis* (1978), whose rich vocabulary and analytical and methodological tools have been immensely useful for my analysis of AIDS. I believe that the AIDS crisis and its construction by the media share some structural resemblances to the mugging phenomenon explored in *Policing the Crisis*. Following that book, I have suggested in chapter 4 that the problem of curing AIDS must be examined partly from a conjuncturalist perspective. It must be viewed as a social and political phenomenon, as an effect of articulation.

In an important reading of the theoretical developments in cultural studies, Lawrence Grossberg (1990) identifies a moment within the history of the Centre for Contemporary Cultural Studies that helps to locate the emergence of the theory of articulation from that history. Defined, rightly, as "structural-conjunctural," the moment refers to the Centre's shift away from both a humanist and a structuralist conception of culture and ideology to a position that, as Grossberg puts it, "changes the rules of the game" (p. 136). The position offers a focused rereading of Gramsci's work as it intersects Williams's humanism and Althusser's structuralism. Although the result—broadly termed "conjuncturalism"—has often been identified as a middle ground between the two, I believe it is positioned closer to Williams than to Althusser. Conjuncturalism strongly retains the notion of (historical) correspondences, while it seeks to incorporate the notion of difference. It agrees with the Althusserean view of culture as a structure built on difference, yet it is reluctant to give up the significance of "tendentiality," of material and historical specificities that give culture its distinctive shape at a given conjuncture. Ideological domination (defined mostly in relation to the notion of consensus), it argues, "prescribes . . . the limits within which ideas and conflicts move and are resolved" (Clark et al., 1975, p. 39). Grossberg writes: "Conjuncturalism argues that while there are no necessary correspondences (relations), there are always real (effective) correspondences" (1990, p. 136).

In conjuncturalism, a theory of difference is thus subsumed under a theory of specificity. This implies that while conjuncturalism follows Althusser's description of the social formation as a "structure in dominance," it insists that it be historicized; while it realizes the importance of "overdetermination," it nonetheless seeks to locate "determinateness" within real historical relations, conditions, and specific tendential lines of force; while it values the "autonomy" of cultural agents and their practices, it demands that it be conceived as relative autonomy. All of this indicates the strength of conjuncturalism, for it seeks to ground culture appropriately in the broader, located, and effect-ive processes of history. The effectivity of *textual* practices depends on how they are positioned within a *contextual* trajectory, the emphasis being shifted from "effect" to "effectivity." What constitutes meaning is not only the effect of the organization of the moments of production and consumption of signs, but also their organicity—the way they are woven into the web of signification chains, their inscription into the dynamic currency of enduring social discourses. Articulation thus aims at an analysis that is longer term, perhaps more accumulative, than that of encoding/decoding.[2]

The theory of articulation emerged from this conjuncturalist position, underscored first by a rejection of a full poststructuralist affirmation of endless difference and second by a deeply political—and rigorously moral—pursuit of a democratic socialism. The term "conjuncturalism" suggests the process of assembling and reassembling positions (intellectual, moral, and social), of converging closures, however temporary. To have a conjuncture is to form a frontier, a temporary fixity of sociopolitical relations that is constantly open for explorations, struggles, and rearticulations. Although this quality of openness can be compared to language, as poststructuralist theories do, this must be done metaphorically, not literally. Hall argues that the antireductionist impulse of poststructuralism has led to a view of society as a totally open discursive field, through a powerfully "literal" equation of the social with language.

> While the metaphor of language is the best way of rethinking many fundamental questions, there's a kind of slippage from acknowledging its utility and power to saying that that's really the way it is. . . . That often becomes its own kind of reductionism. I would say that the fully discur-

sive position is a reductionism upward, rather than a reductionism downward, as economism was. What seems to happen is that, in the reaction against a crude materialism, the metaphor of x operates like y is reduced to x = y. (Hall, quoted in Grossberg, 1986, p. 57)

Hall has the question of ideology in mind as he criticizes such a fully open position that, in his view, tends to destroy altogether the role ideology plays in social struggles. Articulatory practices are made impossible and indeed irrelevant once the social is collapsed into totally free-floating discursive elements. [Or, as Laclau and Mouffe have it, once "the social" has disappeared as a possible analytical or political category (1985, p. 112).] The notion of resistance is also difficult to retain when the question of the constitution of dominance in ideology has been eliminated. In Hall's view, the relations of power cannot be effectively assessed without first conceptualizing the social as a "formation," or without first establishing struggle as the positively sustaining work of coupling and uncoupling meanings (Grossberg, 1986, pp. 48-49; Hall, 1985, pp. 92-93). Articulation is therefore the actualization of ideology and the conduit for the establishment of the social formation (the social *as* formation). It insists on thinking difference "conditionally."

I prefer to think of this necessarily conditional character of difference—which Hall calls "unity-in-difference"—as a frontier, connoting a temporarily built terrain at a given time, connecting and converging diverse resources into an imaginary but effect-ive site. Frontier also bespeaks the possibility for struggle, because it embodies the possibility for renewal and change. At a broad level, therefore, frontier can be thought of in conjunction with a theory of structural (not structuralist) determination. History depends on the enactment of frontiers; the dynamics of historical transformations turn on the dynamics of frontier politics. Understanding history in terms of the setting of limits, the marking of the parameter and space of operation, rather than in terms of the absolute predictability or unpredictability of particular outcomes (that is, necessary correspondence or necessarily no correspondence), is the basis of the theory of articulation, and indeed of a philosophy of conjuncturalism.

Thinking in terms of frontier does not oppose the concept of difference and the radical utility that it allows. The concept of frontier can be used in conjunction with the poststructuralist concept of "field." In Laclau and Mouffe's eloquent poststructuralist rereading of Marxist theory, they use "field of discursivity" to describe the character of the social terrain (1985, p. 111). According to them, the concept of "field" indicates the vast proliferation—indeed, "surpluses"—of differences that render a final closure impossible. How, then, is the concept of field (as a concept of impossibility) consistent with the concept of frontier (as a concept of possibility)? It is important to note that while Laclau and Mouffe insist on the impossibility of any final fixity of meaning, they also remind us of a crucial condition that is necessary for theorizing such an impossibility:

> The impossibility of an ultimate fixity of meaning implies that there have to be partial fixations—otherwise, the very flow of differences would be impossible. Even in order to differ, to subvert meaning, there has to be *a* meaning. . . . Any discourse is constituted as an attempt to dominate the field of discursivity, to arrest the flow of differences, to construct a center. We will call the privileged discursive points of this partial fixation, *nodal points*. (P. 112)

In other words, if we accept the incomplete character of the field of discursivity, we are indeed affirming a dimension of relationality of every identity that differs from another within that field. Frontier is precisely an index of that relationality; it is a nodal point in the vast field of "relational differences." The concept of nodal points is useful for, and not inconsistent with, the theory of articulation.

The images of frontier and field, of course, suggest a language of warfare that characterizes the theory of articulation. No nodal points are ever fixed; they have to be fought for and positively sustained by specific processes. They are not eternal; they constantly have to be renewed, rearticulated. History can be seen as the effect of a complex unity underscored by fixities that are temporary but always powerful, relatively autonomous but always determinate, tendential but always specifically directive. Thus, frontier politics only becomes effective if it connects with a particular constellation of social forces in the field—a battle over hegemonic power in a specific space and time. It also crystallizes one of the central Marxist maxims that has informed Hall's work: people make history, but in conditions not of their making. There are always possibilities of struggle, but they always take place within and over a concretely contested terrain.

This spirit guided one of the most important contributions of cultural studies: the study of the conditions of racism in *Policing the Crisis* (Hall et al., 1978). This book presents an immensely useful model for applying the theory of articulation to media studies. In Grossberg's description of the development of cultural studies, he has suggested that *Policing the Crisis* represents the first real sign of the increasing pull of Gramscian conjuncturalism, shifting the study of ideology to

> a greater emphasis on popular languages and common sense, on the construction of a field of meanings and differences which is linked, on the one hand, to hegemonic projects and, on the other, to certain conditions of possibility. (1990, p. 135)

I have employed this important work as a reference, attempting to adhere to its theoretical principles.

*Policing the Crisis* is a detailed investigation of the peculiarly massive response of the media, the judiciary system, and the general public to a robbery—labeled a mugging—committed in Handsworth, England, in 1972. The case was peculiar because, although the crime was familiar to London streets from at least the 1860s, it was described by the press and the police as "a frightening new strain of crime." Debates sprang up over what this "new" crime meant. In a short time, the debates had led to a renewed panic over an apparent growing tide of violence, an apparent breakdown of the moral fabric of the British way of life, and an apparent softening or even collapse of British law and order. Such perceptions justified an escalation of crime-control measures. By 1976, such debates seemed to have condensed around a single effective "origin": black youth in the inner city. By then, mugging and blacks had become synonymous terms in the public imagination.

All of this transformed the Handsworth event into a phenomenon contained in the signifier "mugging." The fear around the Handsworth case grew into a fear of something much larger, much more menacing; the social control of such fear therefore became much more severe, much more "justifiable." Taking a skeptical view of this constructed "newness" of such crime, the authors of *Policing the Crisis* suggest that the analysis of the Handsworth case unearths a whole terrain of contested forces, shaping the incident from outside, behind the scenes, and linked to a certain hegemonic struggle for the power of the state to step up control, not of the crime per se but of the social group thought to be unmistakably associated with the crime: the black youth.

*Policing the Crisis* actuates the theory by relocating the study of ideology from a transactional to a structural and historical model of analysis.

The authors clarify their aim in a passage that sets the terms of their analysis:

> This book aims to go behind the label [mugging] to the contradictory social content which is mystifyingly reflected in it: but it is *not* a book about why certain individuals, as individuals, turn to mugging; nor about what practical steps can be taken to control or reduce its incidence; nor about how awful a crime "mugging" is. . . . We *are* concerned with "mugging"—but as a social phenomenon, rather than as a particular form of street crime. . . . Once you perceive "mugging" not as a fact but as a relation—the relation between crime and the reaction to crime—the conventional wisdoms about "mugging" fall apart in your hands. If you look at this relation in terms of the social forces and the contradictions accumulating within it (rather than simply in terms of the danger to ordinary folks), or in terms of the wider historical context in which it occurs (i.e., in terms of a historical conjuncture, not just a date on the calendar), the whole terrain of the problem changes in character. (Hall et al., 1978, vii-viii; emphasis in the original)

The historical issues, they argue, are precisely the "critical forces which *produce* 'mugging' in the specific form in which it appears" (p. 185; emphasis in the original). They remind us that crime, like all other events, is a social and historical, not a "natural," phenomenon. The Handsworth case crystallizes the operation of the media, so that through one case we can observe the shape of a whole news process and its relation to hegemony. The theory of articulation offers a useful vantage point from which to consider a historical phenomenon such as mugging and the role that the legal institutions play in the attempt to maintain the stability and cohesion of society through the (hyper)control of crime. *Policing the Crisis* discovered a repressed terrain of discourses, attitudes, and practices against blacks, all of which predated the Handsworth case, and in many significant ways determined how the incident was interpreted and how it was then "appropriately" responded to, contained, and policed.

In *Policing the Crisis*, the authors specify the way in which the media are critically connected to the world beyond—the context beyond the text—and the way in which such a connection orchestrates together with the ruling ideas of the time. The authors stress that the "fit" between the news media and the ruling ideas is rooted in the institutional connections between them. They suggest that the routine structure of news production relies on (1) the regular supply of "pre-scheduled events" by institutional sources and (2) the journalistic codes of objectivity and impartiality, themselves institutionally produced rules. These two factors combine to produce "a systematically structured *over-accessing* to the media of those in powerful and privileged institutional positions" (p. 58). This does not necessarily mean a wholesale delivery of institutionally privileged ideas, but the media has nonetheless entered into a position of structured subordination to the primary sources/definers of society.

One specific way in which the articulation of cultural identities is realized is in the use of the feature story. Feature stories are *"inherently* ideological, for what they seek to do is to contextualize the event, place it in the social world" (p. 96). They signal a movement from the surface of the event (the problem, the dilemma) to its underlying root (the cause, the motivation, the backdrop), and by doing so draw on a wider field of discourse, which is then offered up as the "true and in-depth explanation" of the event. The insertion of the event into a larger map of the social and ideological world is often the mechanism by which the nodal point of discourse is formed. Such a contextualization can be achieved through at least two concrete means.

The first is the extensive use of biographical details of those who are involved in the event, as victim or as perpetrator (pp. 96-97). These details are usually obtained from professional experts, from local connections (friends, relatives, neighbors), and from the individuals implicated in the event. The biographical details suggest that there is more to the event than meets the eye; the individuals who are documented now have a history, their actions an explainable "origin." This process also helps journalists to construct a locale, or more specifically an image of a locale, within which the individuals and their actions acquire a typographical relation to the story. In *Policing the Crisis*, the authors find that one of the most powerful ways by which the Handsworth case acquires its spectacular ideological power is through feature stories' construction of an "image of decay," offered as the single effective *spectacle* of mugging. Analysis is collapsed into image; concrete investigation is replaced by generalized analogy. Such a strategy generates a series of "transcendent" associations based on the journalists' reading of biographical information of black youth: inner-city ghettos, past records of street fights, siblings or parents previously involved in criminal activities, low-income housing, unstable family backgrounds, unemployment, and so on. Finally, there is a terrain, a subaltern ghetto, that can be presented to the "general public."

The second method of contextualization is the use of "montage effect" and "microcosm effect" (p. 105). The montage effect refers to the way feature stories arrange and examine competing values and worldviews about the background elements of a case side by side. It conveys an impression of comprehensiveness and balance. The microcosm effect refers to the way the general background themes are distilled and condensed into a local instance, invested with opposing opinions from the local community. These opposing opinions are also set against each other. What the montage and microcosm effects achieve is an "endorsement" of particular (selected) interpretations without actively trying to privilege one over the other. Ideological inflections have been suggested; they just appear in many faces. The feature stories thus manage to firm up their formal appearance of breadth, depth, and balance at the same time.

Once articulation has been established in the media, it produces a context and a "control response." As a product of articulation, the context therefore contains not only the elements that constitute its presence, but also the elements that support or sustain its legitimacy. In *Policing the Crisis,* for instance, the journalistic explanations of mugging not only successfully transform mugging into a discourse about a sustained upsurge of violence and moral degeneration, they also marshal an authoritarian consensus toward a hyperdisciplinary state. The connection between articulation and hegemony is forged; together they are the dual pathway of control, from the formation of a realizable and objectivized frontier to the materialization of concrete domination as it is legitimized by the construction of the policing and policed subjects.

In the context of a discourse theory and a conjuncturalist theory, the ubiquitous problem of "curing" AIDS presides over semiotic, discursive, and "frontier" relations that, through amazing leaps and bounces, recharge not only technomedical cultures, but the historical epoch in which we now live. To further think through the importance assumed by curing as a phantasmic preoccupation, I offer a few useful interpretive signposts whose aim is to forge some openings that erupt, inevitably, from the closure of a book.

## Some Theoretical Axioms of "Curing"

### Curing is grounded in the historical fields of health and life sciences

The cultural history of health and life sciences forms the crucial background from which we may locate the emphasis on curing. The development of health and life sciences must be conceptualized on the basis of the technologies of power that are contemporary with it. As Foucault (1984) has argued, modernization—and the power that accompanies it—was firmly grounded in the development and rigorous expansion of the social fields of knowledge that were centrally concerned with averting all imminent threats to people's lives. Such fields of knowledge included agricultural development; nutrition science; systems to monitor and control mortality and morbidity; welfare and housing development; and, of course, modern medicine. Diseases, disasters, and death were perceived as antithetical to the entire discourse of modernization. More important, they drew attention to the limits of power: "Death is power's limit, the moment that escapes it" (Foucault, 1984, p. 261).

By inversion, it was over life—its processes of survival and maintenance—that power established its domination. Power replaced the fear of the inevitability and sometimes randomness of death (as a result of diseases and disasters) by a systematic and positive production of a discourse with an unchallengeable aim: the aim of preserving life. This discourse did not merely serve to avert the morbid, unpleasant attention to death, it functioned as the material effect of power practiced over the body. Throughout Foucault's work, he has argued that this power over life has evolved largely in two forms: the procedures of disciplines (focused on the extortion and integration of the body's forces—and docility—into systems of efficient and economic controls) and the technologies of reproduction (focused on the regulations of and interventions into the spheres of sexuality, health, expectancy, and longevity). According to Foucault, the organization of the power over life was deployed around these two discourses (1984, p. 262). Thus, for power to take hold of the body, it first had to designate the necessity of health—the basic right to life—as an existential ideal, as the concrete essence of being, as the realization of the possible, and most important, as a pressure to justify the benefits thought to have been brought about by modernization.

What was a general theme regarding biological existence became a meticulous science imbued with political implications. The articulation of power over the body therefore rested upon the moral, historical, and political ideal that attempted to ensure the welfare, maintenance, and survival of the body. With this, death had been perceived as more and more unacceptable, not because of its essential morbidness, but because of its threat to social productivity. The preservation of life, and the desire to avoid the subject of death whenever possible, can therefore be seen as a political hegemony achieved in the name of economic interests and the ethics of health. Historically, in the United States this emphasis on health can be said to have constituted a "Right to Life" movement, which can be seen, among other places, in the War on Cancer campaign, the anti-smoking campaigns, and the systematic development and proliferation of popular health education, including education about dietary and fitness controls. Underlying this Right to Life movement is the shining furrow of medicine's authority.

We must situate the politics of curing within this historical discourse that places the practices and ideologies of a particular vision of health at its center. If health is no longer conceptualized as a random or natural substrate of life but as a discourse that passes into power's sphere of control, then it is hardly surprising that curing arises as the designated ideal in the social and scientific discussion of treatment issues surrounding a disease. The power to invest life through and through makes curing one of the noblest pursuits of modern sciences. The Right to Life movement in recent Western history described by Foucault can be seen as the pretext of the contemporary discourse of curing, surrounded by the same power of discipline and regulation of the body.

*Curing rests upon the semiotic relations to health, life, disease, and death*

In order for curing to have become a master code in the language of AIDS treatment, it, like any code, rests upon the play of differences. We may say that a cure is disease's difference. A disease contaminates, "leaks," signifies breaking in or breaking down. A cure rejuvenates, purifies, restores control. A cure is also death's difference, one more profound and totalizing than that which differentiates disease from death. "From the point of view of death, disease has a land, a mappable territory, a subter-ranean" (Foucault, 1975, p. 149). In other words, death unleashes the narrative of the living and the healthy. For not only must death be death (a matter too important to be banal), it must be death in relation to the antideath. The desire for life and health plays on their semantic and material difference from death. Particularly, health promises a place far-thest from death, a land specified by the prospect of the cure.

The cure therefore offers the fantasy of the antideath; it seduces an imagination of immortality. It is a mode of defense, a disavowal of the traumatic and the mysterious. The more the spectacles of disease and death are displayed (as they are displayed in the discourse of AIDS), and the more deeply the anxiety attached to these events begins to circulate among us, the deeper the desire for the cure. The emergence of the discourse of curing as a condensed category seems to be the result of the emergence of serialized binary identities about the body: health/disease, disease/death, death/life, life/cure, cure/health. This logic of antithesis enables and legitimizes whatever it takes to find "the cure." It thus may limit the treatment strategies that do not conform to dichotomous definitions of wellness and illness.

Conceptualized as both a semiotic of differences and a historical discourse of the body, curing becomes a crucial political object of knowledge/power. The fact of "being cured" therefore has deep political implications. Curing is no longer just a fact of social and medical endeavor; instead it is the crucial articulator of power's intervention into the material body on the basis of a historical discourse that enables the far-reaching importance assumed by the technologies of lifesaving. We may say that the intensely *moral* character assumed by curing is the outcome of this *political* context. Power speaks of and to curing; the latter is not a matter of random focus, it is a chosen object and target.

*Curing creates hierarchies of social identities and bodies according to health status and the perception of "risk"*

The power to turn curing into a dominant social priority partly concerns the imagination of the purified body. By now, "purification" is a familiar theme in the discussion of potential AIDS treatments.[3] The identification of curing and purifying emerges from its obverse: the historical identification of disease and filth (see Brandt, 1987). The "plague model" used to describe AIDS since the early years of the epidemic is partly based on this collective fantasy of dualism. The massive press commentary on how the epidemic ravages large sections of the population has intensified the antithesis between disease and filth on the one hand, and curing and purification on the other.

But what is curable and purifiable depends on *who* is perceived to be curable and purifiable according to the highly innovative and authoritative language of "risk." The perception of riskiness can be deceiving. Although everyone is at risk with HIV infection, the cultural categorization of people into normal/abnormal (read: pure/impure) social groups in turn recategorizes them into nonrisky and risky groups, respectively. A social identity purports to shield one from risk (a cultural perception), even though one's behavior may put one at risk (a medical reality).

Conversely, a perceived abnormal identity presupposes risk, even though one may not engage in risky behavior.

In a peculiar way, the discourse of curing may be linked with the discourse of risk. The symbolic stratifications of normal/abnormal and pure/impure—which imply nonriskiness/riskiness—also presuppose curability/incurability (not the actual status of being cured or not, but the different social and political treatment accorded to individuals who seek medical attention). The fantasy link made between symbolic categories of identities creates profound confusion with the behavioral cause of the disease and has a determining effect on people's treatment experience. The experience of curing is not immune from that wicked by-product of prejudice, the stigmatization of identities.

Accordingly, a multiplicity of differences has emerged that produces peculiar types of stratifications upon which the moralistic politics of AIDS treatment is accented. A typology of identities has been built within those relations of difference, and social groups can be separated along such differences. The typology does not only demarcate "us" from "them"—an essentialism that (still) accompanies every aspect of the discourse of AIDS—it also constructs categories of difference within each side, elevating our anxiety over who is healthy/pure/not risky/curable and who is sick/impure/risky/incurable. In table 4, I attempt to make sense of the logic of these symbolic stratifications by charting all the possible combinations of identities implicated in the grid. Imaginary names of people will be used as examples of the different social groups.

The articulation of the problematic category of risk into the healthy/sick axis suddenly creates an explosion of comparisons, in addition to the already-existing divisions based on perceived health status. In table 4, I assume four basic (simplified) types of perceptions that can be created when the factors of health statuses and risk are meshed together. The stratifications of identities (and bodies) can occur both externally among the four types of perceptions (e.g., the differentiation between Terence and Alice) and internally within each type (e.g., Terence and Sarah). In the table, I have only indicated one example of comparison that can occur in each stratification. I do not imagine that society differentiates among the healthy who are also perceived as members of the nonrisk groups (e.g., uninfected adult heterosexual men like Peter, or uninfected children like Alice). Within this scheme of difference, this group is thought to occupy no space in the world of curing. Their present healthiness and their presumed "normality" require no curing; they are the pro-

Table 4. Symbolic stratifications of health, sickness, and "risk"

*Perception 1: Healthy but in risk group*
Terence: uninfected gay man
Sarah: uninfected hemophiliac

*Perception 2: Healthy and in nonrisk group*
Peter: uninfected heterosexual
Alice: uninfected child

*Perception 3: Sick and in risk group*
Paul: gay man with HIV symptoms
Ryan: hemophiliac with HIV symptoms

*Perception 4: Sick but in nonrisk group*
Kim: infected heterosexual with HIV symptoms
Nick: infected child with HIV symptoms

|  | The healthy (risk group) | The healthy (nonrisk group) | The sick (risk group) | The sick (nonrisk group) |
|---|---|---|---|---|
| The healthy (risk group) | Sarah vs. Terence | Terence vs. Alice | Sarah vs. Ryan | Terence vs. Kim |
| The healthy (nonrisk group) | Peter vs. Sarah | No stratification | Alice vs. Ryan | Peter vs. Kim |
| The sick (risk group) | Paul vs. Terence | Paul vs. Peter | No stratification | Ryan vs. Kim |
| The sick (nonrisk group) | Nick vs. Sarah | Nick vs. Alice | Nick vs. Paul | Kim vs. Nick |

totype of the "pure bodies" against which all other bodies are to be measured. At the other extreme, no differentiation is thought necessary for the sick who are also perceived as members of the risk groups (e.g., symptomatic gays like Paul, drug users, or male and female prostitutes). They would represent the prototype of the impure bodies, closely identified with the incurable bodies. They "belong" firmly to the disease side of the disease/cure equation. In effect, this extreme "sickness," situated at the bottom of the hierarchy of identities, encourages a premature death sentence, foreclosing all possibility of survival or of being cured.

Assuming that stratifications occur both externally and internally, I imagine assembling the minimum number of individuals from the four categories of perception (e.g., eight individuals), and we then end up with fourteen possible relations. But when each individual is compared to the rest based on the fourteen relations, we in fact have many more combinations of differences (possibly more than eighty). The peculiar mathematics of relations create not only the divisive stratifications of people's identities and bodies, they also set in motion a culture of anxiety. The imagination of our "curability" is nonetheless tainted by this plethora of multiple but binarized relations, causing further unnecessary fear and stigmatization.

No difference of disease/death and disease/cure is not, at the same time, the difference of bodies. Every body is rendered a negating body; it is always a third-person body, located in others. One's health status, one's chance of surviving the disease or of being cured, now constructed as medical and sociobehavioral entities, are forever shifting: always more and always less than the next person in the complex system of stratifications. The (imaginary) hierarchies inscribe everyone in the anxiety-provoking world of us/them, risk/nonrisk, visible symptom/invisible illness. Despite all the earnestness in the world, the work of curing AIDS is implicated in this anxiety machine.

*Curing invokes a cultural desire for an imaginary "ending" akin to a narrative closure*

A theoretical consideration of curing must incorporate a consideration of narrativity, defined as a textual entity with structured moments in narrative progression. Scientific and historical accounts, like fictional ones, have narrative structures that give order to phenomena.[4] In the context of the theoretical perspective assumed in this book, if AIDS is to be considered a (multiple) narrative created by the media and scientific discourses, then, like any traditional narrative, it inevitably anticipates an ending or a closure. And, like all other moments of the narrative, its ending has to be imagined, manufactured, and circulated. An analogy can therefore be drawn between narrative ending and curing. For just as the search for a cure drives scientific research toward the desired end point where the disease is thought to have been "controlled" or even "stopped," an ending carries the similar driving force within a narrative movement toward a point of finality.

Endings are always speculative; they embody the future, the probable, and the unknown. But as a culturally envisioned possibility, an ending is essential—and seductive—for the AIDS story; it provides the closure expected of a traditional narrative. Although any definition of the end of a crisis is somewhat arbitrary (as arbitrary as, say, the "end of the Vietnam War," the "end of the cold war," or the "end of communism"), the desire for a narrative and psychological closure is powerful, especially in the case of the AIDS crisis.

To think in terms of ending is not to displace the present critical condition by wishful thinking or to dilute its immediacy. On the contrary, it puts the present in a wider geography of history by which we may be able to map the present more clearly. One may even argue that to understand

AIDS at all, we need to examine how its imagined ending is culturally conceived and politically deployed. If a cure for AIDS has not been found yet, it has to be (culturally) invented. The desire for a cure is therefore the seduction of narrative control. As I mentioned in previous chapters, curing (as a matter of medical care) and controlling (as a matter of power) are frequently inseparable.

In telling the AIDS story, the media is caught in a complex web of social and medical discourses that precedes, and subsequently structures, the AIDS story. And, as the media is also caught up in the powerful impulse toward constructing a foreseeable, controllable narrative closure for the AIDS story, it reproduces the contradictory definitions of curability/incurability. Loaded down with cultural, psychological, and political baggage, the problem of "curing AIDS" goes far beyond the control of the disease itself.

### Curing is an analytic internal to the logic of temporality

Consider the following brief exchange reported by Joel Davis, a freelance science writer for popular science magazines in the United States, which took place between himself and Richard Thorne, a scientist at Cambridge BioScience, a small biotechnology firm in Hopkinton, Massachusetts:

> "How far away *are* we from an AIDS vaccine, do you think?" I asked.
> Thorne shook his head. "It's hard to make that kind of prediction. It would mean you can foresee all the problems. This is a case where there are no existing solutions to some of the very fundamental problems. New knowledge is necessary. How do you predict when new knowledge comes up?
> "We can say this: *It's not forever*. A lot of very bright people are working on an AIDS vaccine, and *it will happen*. But it is hard to put a time frame on it." Thorne looked at me. "It may be sooner than a lot of people realize." (Davis, 1989, p. 197; emphasis in the original)

Like Davis, all of us have at some point been anxious to know the secrets of technomedical science, so that we may acquire an ascriptive security of knowing something now, in the certifiable present, and to ask "How far away are we from a cure for AIDS?" The question is, after all, peculiar in its casting of a temporal-mathematical query: the "cure" appears as an object in a projected temporal distance, like a banana to a caged, hungry monkey. The answer must therefore measure the temporal distance between the present and a presumably knowable future (presumed, that is, by the question itself), between the cage and a reachable banana. But this desire "to know now" is only a double textual foil that defers twice. First, "to know now" inevitably generates "to know the future," and thus establishes the supremacy of the future as the keeper of the secret. "To know the future" just as surely generates, in Davis's (and our) inquiry, its intended object: the scientist who intercedes between "to know now" and "to know the future." Second, "to know now" in fact means "can't know now," a moment of a failure of prediction, a failure to foresee: "It's hard to make that kind of prediction. It would mean you can foresee all the problems." Yet "can't know now" inevitably generates, in Thorne's answer, its intended effect: the recuperation of an authority to prophesize an indefinite definity—"It's not forever"; "it will happen." We must note that "it" here refers to a highly ambivalent subject: "new knowledge"? Or a "cure"?

In this series of textual deferments of time, a time map used for a discourse about the "cure" is constructed by the scientist: new knowledge, not cure, can and will be attainable at any point between now and forever, if the sanctity of this temporal order is kept inviolate. This time map renders our anxious question—"How far away are we from an AIDS cure?"—meaningless; the least illuminating point from which to ask this question is the present. Our entrapment in the present and our anxious desire to know now, like the hungry monkey trapped in the cage, has guided us to an elusive target: our desire for a "cure." For it is clear that, according to the scientist's time map, the "real" secret is time itself, whose spectacular performances would deliver us out of misery—performances such as the ability of time to paralyze the present, to place supremacy in the future, to manufacture "new knowledge," and to render itself invisible by casting the elusive target of the "cure."

Thorne's irresolute response now appears to be a vehicle to masquerade a deeper sense of certainty rooted in the mastery of time. The "cure," if cure there be, must therefore be understood as an analytic internal to time's logic. The banana isn't the solution to the caged monkey's hunger; the realization of the stick nearby, which must be aligned properly in the space between the cage and the fruit, is what would eventually "cure."

In the unknowing present moment that we occupy—a moment of inevitable opacity—and under a technostructure whose experts tell us they "don't know" but "it" will happen, a whole discursive machinery by which the knowledge about "curing" AIDS gets constructed is trundled into our field of vision. We educate ourselves about the reality of

HIV infection through the temporal metaphors of "life cycle" and "time bomb." We educate ourselves about the gruesome reality of what would happen to our bodies in HIV/AIDS, again through temporal constructs such as "living on borrowed time" and "developmental symptomatic stages." We sign up for clinical drug trials organized around time tables we don't understand but must comply with. We read the horrific projections of AIDS deaths in the *New York Times* and listen to them on CNN. And in the most heightened moment of our present state of unknowingness, we learn, the moment a person receives a seropositive test result, what it all means, again through the temporal discourse vindictively captured in such dictums as "AIDS is invariably fatal" and "AIDS Kills Fags Dead." By this process, we learn about our powerlessness, unless we can finally conquer the inconquerable wall of time.

And we, as an alert people in the crisis, see that the sovereignty of time over our bodies and our consciousness in fact spins out and is spun from a series of (old) dilemmas: the dichotomy of "the expert" and "the patient," the dependence on and resistance to organized medicine, the spectacular confusion over AZT's usefulness, the ideological juxtaposition of health status and risk status, the psychic schism between surviving (guiltily) and dying (unnecessarily), and, most of all, the cracking definition of AIDS as both curable (controlled/contained) and incurable (morbid/menace).

Among all of us who are witnessing the course of development of the AIDS crisis, the way we preside over the constructions of the possibilities of "curing" AIDS—anxiously, angrily, passively, longingly, energetically, remorsefully, skeptically, quietly, depressingly, numbly, guiltily, confusingly, indifferently, or some or all of the above—significantly defines our political relation to our homophobic and savage culture, our social relation with one another, and our mortal relation with our own well-being. I do not assume that to develop an analytical shield around such a reality, as I have chosen to do in this book, is a more innocuous process, for either gay or nongay readers, or for those deeply affected or those yet untouched by AIDS, than the process of confronting it with our instinct and natural passion. Nor do I assume that a serious and systematic consideration of the question of "curing" AIDS—as I have chosen for my project with, all along, a contradictory desire to disavow it and to be seduced by it—would necessarily be more illuminating of the present disposition of our society, culture, and history transformed by AIDS than a focus on other issues in the crisis. The threat of AIDS in many developing countries, the exponential increase of the number of women from all walks of life being infected with HIV, or the realization by more and more scientists that HIV may not be a sufficient cause for AIDS are only a few of the urgent realities that also require our attention.

I do assume, pessimistically, that the moment of the "End of AIDS" brought about by a "cure" in its multiple, combined forms—or by some other visions and practices of healing outside the paradigm of "curing"— would not end the savage and brutal fantasies and actions directed at the oppressed that the AIDS crisis has painfully revealed. More optimistically, I know that such a moment will be filled with so much jubilation for all of us that we will go on celebrating in our most fabulous selves and leave books like this on the shelves to gather dust.

# Appendix: A Summary of the Major Treatment-Related Stories Reported on Network Television News, 1985-1992

In this Appendix, which draws upon the Vanderbilt Television News Archive in Nashville, Tennessee, I provide a chronological synopsis of the television networks' (ABC, CBS, NBC) news coverage of AIDS treatment activities, highlighting the moments that constitute the discourse of curing AIDS. Individuals and organizations associated with AIDS treatment are named to familiarize readers with the central players of the discourse.

I have included in this chronology the related coverage that began before 1987, the year that I suggest as the inaugurating moment for the discourse of "curing" AIDS. I believe that the events that took place before the FDA's approval of AZT in 1987 provide crucial background information for understanding the events that followed.

*July to September 1985:* Numerous reports speculate over Rock Hudson's mysterious illness and his secret travel to Paris for treatment by a drug known as HPA-23. Reactions to the drug from U.S. researchers were skeptical, especially from the National Cancer Institute's (NCI) Sam Broder (who was vigorously testing another drug, AL-721, at the time). French researchers defended the drug's potential usefulness. There were also reports of new calls for more research funding for the test of another experimental drug, Suramin.

*September 1985*: ABC news offered a five-part series called "AIDS: Facts and Fears" from September 23 to 27. Part 4 dealt with drug treatment issues; attention was given to five drugs being tested at the time: Suramin, Foscarnet, Compound S (AZT), Ribavirin, and HPA-23. Scientists William Haseltine of the Dana-Farber Cancer Institute and Harvard Medical School, Robert Gallo of the National Cancer Institute, and Broder explained difficulties in developing treatment. A person with AIDS (PWA), Kerry Shapiro, acknowledged the odds against his survival.

*October and November 1985:* First reports of an AIDS-related drug, Cyclosporine A; controversy revolved around U.S. researchers' skeptical reactions to this French-developed drug. French researchers were accused of spreading premature publicity of the drug's potential efficacy. Deaths from the drug were reported.

*November 14, 1985:* CBS news gave the first report of testing of Compound S (later known as AZT). Sam Broder, David Ho, and a patient, John Solomon, were interviewed. Solomon was to appear often in later treatment-related reports.

*June 22-25, 1986:* All three networks aired a total of six reports on the Second International Conference on AIDS held in Paris. The reports offered very little discussion of treatment research, giving attention to (1) the dispute between France and the United States over the patent right to HIV; (2) the scientists' attempt to establish a reliable global epidemiology; and (3) the increasing anxiety over the spread of AIDS to the heterosexual population (a great deal of air time was devoted to AIDS in Africa, where it was determined that the disease was spread primarily through heterosexual contact).

*December 1985 to March 1987:* Seventeen reports on AZT oscillated between optimism and skepticism toward the drug. The June 30, 1986, report by ABC news discussed the debate between Mathilde Krim (American Foundation for AIDS Research, or AmFAR) and Burroughs Wellcome's David Barry over the ethics of the clinical trials method. AZT's side effects were frequently emphasized. Experts repeatedly shown included physicians Paul Volberding of San Francisco General Hospital, Broder, and Krim, and Burroughs Wellcome spokespersons; patients repeatedly interviewed included John Solomon and Jon Stewart.

*January 9, 1987:* ABC news gave the first report of Ribavirin as a potential AIDS-fighting drug. This and two other reports about the drug (May 27, 1987, on CBS; March 21, 1988, on NBC) focused on how the drug was illegally smuggled from Mexico, and the charges made by the medical community that the drug company, ICN Pharmaceuticals, had proclaimed success prematurely and thereby reaped profit from stock-market gain.

*January 27, 1987:* ABC news reported a statement made by the surgeon general, C. Everett Koop, that a cure for AIDS would never be found. Koop also appeared on NBC's "Face the Nation" on March 29, where he expressed pessimism that an AIDS vaccine would be developed by the end of the century.

*March to May 1987 :* Many reports detailed the Food and Drug Administration's (FDA) effort to ease government regulations on experimental drugs, including relaxing testing requirements and allowing patients wider access to unapproved drugs. At the same time, numerous reports focused on the development of the underground AIDS drug networks.

*March 20, 1987:* Government approval of AZT was announced by all three networks. Praises were noted by scientists (Broder, Anthony Fauci of the National Institute of Allergy and Infectious Diseases, and Volberding), by Barry of Burroughs Wellcome, and by PWAs John Solomon and Jay Van Horn. Gay Men's Health Crisis (GMHC) spokesperson Tim Sweeney was the first to criticize the high cost of AZT. More extensive reports of the cost debate came a few days later on NBC and CBS news.

*March 27, 1987:* ABC news's "Person of the Week" featured Dr. Jerome Horwitz, who discovered the AZT compound in the 1960s.

*April 1, 1987:* ABC news examined President Reagan's first public address on AIDS. Reagan's speech to the College of Physicians called for abstinence and claimed that the government had put high priority on developing an AIDS cure. Representative Henry Waxman and GMHC's Richard Dunn were shown questioning the credibility of the Reagan administration on the issue.

*May 31-June 5, 1987:* All three networks aired a total of fourteen reports on the Third International Conference on AIDS held in Washington, D.C. About half of the reports focused on the public objection to Reagan's recent announcement about a national mandatory testing program. The other reports focused on the increasing fear among health professionals of infection through caring for AIDS patients. Reports on treatment research spotlighted AZT, because it was newly approved.

*November 12, 1987:* A report by CBS news for the first time distinguished HIV infection from AIDS, noting that infection did not mean full-blown AIDS and that some infected people stayed healthy and alive for a long time.

*June 12-16, 1988:* All three networks aired a total of ten reports on the Fourth International Conference on AIDS held in Stockholm, Sweden. The reports stressed the changing profile of the epidemic, pointing to minorities and infants as the growing risk groups. Continual attention was given to research of HIV's properties and to vaccine experiments. The new concept of combination therapy, particularly the combination of AZT with other drugs such as CD4, was discussed.

*June 17, 1988:* ABC news's "Person of the Week" featured Dan Zagury, a French scientist who injected an experimental vaccine into himself and his staff. Zagury was compared to past scientists who used self-experimentation (Freud's use of cocaine, Fossman's heart research, and Salk's polio vaccine research). Generally, coverage of vaccine research was sporadic; most featured Gallo, who emphasized the difficulty of such research.

*October 11, 1988:* All three networks reported ACT UP's massive protest at FDA headquarters in Rockville, Maryland.

*February 7, 1989:* ABC news's "American Agenda" featured "Medicine: Government and Drugs," a report of the problems of the traditional drug development process and changes in the FDA as a result of pressure from AIDS patients and activists.

*March 14, 1989:* ABC and CBS news reported that HIV could become resistant to AZT after a period of use. It was noted that viruses often learned to elude drugs.

*April 11, 1989:* ABC news aired a special report on "American Agenda" called "Medicine: AIDS Remedies," which examined the development and impact of the "peddling of untested remedies for AIDS." The alternative remedies discussed included spiritual healing and vaccination with typhoid vaccine. Reports of the underground drug networks had been appearing since a CBS report on May 5, 1985.

*April 1989:* CBS and NBC news first reported Compound Q as a possible cure for AIDS, featuring Dr. Michael McGrath as the discoverer of the potential antiviral ability of the Chinese cucumber root in vitro. Commentary centered on the drug's possible side effects, the anxiety expressed by scientists regarding illegal smuggling of Compound Q from

China, the secret trials conducted by Project Inform (a San Francisco-based community organization that develops educational materials about promising therapies for PWAs), and finally the FDA's refusal to comment on the secret trials. On June 26, NBC reported the death of one participant of the trial conducted by Project Inform.

*June 4-8, 1989*: A total of nine reports of the Fifth International Conference on AIDS held in Montreal, Canada, covered for the first time the idea that AIDS had become a "manageable" disease. The central focus of these reports was Salk's vaccine research.

*July 27, 1989*: NBC news first reported the significance of ddI as a useful alternative to AZT. The ddI story was not followed through until March 12, 1990 (ABC, CBS) when several deaths resulting from "unmonitored use" of the drug were reported.

*August 17-18, 1989*: CBS news reported a new development in AZT research that indicated its usefulness for early use by those who were asymptomatic. The August 17 report focused on the experts' view of this new "breakthrough," including that of Louis Sullivan, health and human services secretary; Fauci; Bill Mason, a patient; Volberding; GMHC's Dunn; and Project Inform's Martin Delaney. The August 18 report focused on the response from gay rights groups and patients. The AZT story quickly became an issue of persuading high-risk groups to obtain early testing so as to start AZT treatment before the onset of symptoms.

*November 13, 1989*: ABC news reported the resignation of FDA commissioner Frank Young, who cited public pressure and internal problems in FDA as reasons.

*December 19, 1989*: ABC and CBS news reported some researchers' claim that they had cleared HIV from the bodies of AIDS patients using bone marrow transplants. Both reports included a severe rebuttal by Fauci, who objected to the *New York Times*'s front-page coverage of the findings as premature because the findings were preliminary.

*March 1990*: All three networks reported the beginning of human trials for Jonas Salk's vaccine for AIDS. Also noted was the Catholic church's attempt to recruit elderly priests and nuns as voluntary participants for the trials.

*May 21, 1990*: All three networks reported ACT UP's massive protest at the National Institutes of Health. By now, a visual history of the group's demonstrations was available, complete with dates, representative spokespersons (e.g., Larry Kramer, cofounder of the Gay Men's Health Crisis; activist Mark Harrington), and footage of activists, always encoded as angry, defiant, and rude.

*June 17-24, 1990*: All three networks aired a total of eighteen reports of the Sixth International Conference on AIDS held in San Francisco. The controversy over immigration law barring PWAs from entering the United States dominated the coverage. Reports about treatment development focused on the Salk vaccine and on the new findings regarding Compound Q presented by Project Inform's Delaney. The final reports seemed to suggest a collective conclusion that, as a result of the better-organized AIDS protests at the sites of the conference, future conferences on AIDS would probably not be held in the United States. (Almost everyone realized that the true reason for changing conference sites had to do with the U.S. government's discriminatory immigration policy.)

*January 2-3, 1991*: ABC news's "American Agenda" presented a two-part report on the legal battles surrounding the monopoly of AZT by Burroughs Wellcome.

*May to June 1991*: NBC and CBS covered the "tenth anniversary" of the AIDS crisis. The reports included statistics of AIDS cases, deaths, and research funding, as well as a discussion of future vaccine research. There was a brief discussion of the emerging crisis of AIDS in Asia.

*June 12, 1991*: All three networks covered a report in *New England Journal of Medicine* on the genetic engineering of the HIV that might lead to a vaccine to treat those already infected by the virus. Details were given of research on military volunteers.

*June 14, 1991*: ABC news's "Person of the Week" featured Dr. Jonas Salk. Salk's background was reviewed, and historical scenes of his famous polio vaccine research were shown. Salk's discussion of vaccine research for AIDS was then contrasted with Anthony Fauci's caution about AIDS immunization.

*June 1991*: News from the Seventh International Conference on AIDS, held in Florence, Italy, focused mainly on the research report that HIV could be contracted from kissing. The Centers for Disease Control was reported to recommend against exchange of bodily fluids, including saliva.

*October 9, 1991:* All three networks reported the FDA's approval of the new drug ddI.

*March 10, 1992:* NBC reported the U.S. Public Health Service's announcement that most patients suffering from AIDS, glaucoma, and cancer would not be allowed to use marijuana to ease their suffering.

*April 1992:* NBC news compared the relative advantages of AZT, ddI, and ddC (ddC being close to FDA approval).

*July 17-25, 1992:* All three networks covered the Eighth International Conference on AIDS, held in Amsterdam, The Netherlands. The breaking news was about the "mystery virus," hypothesized to be a new strain of HIV that could not be detected by current tests. An increase in the discussion of women with AIDS and the link between AIDS and tuberculosis was evident in the coverage. The question of the "mystery virus" continued to capture the networks' attention in the following months.

# Notes

## Introduction

1. This exercise is inspired by Paula Treichler's brilliant essay (1992a) on the cultural construction of HIV and AIDS, in which she unpacks the apodictic claim "HIV causes AIDS" to reveal a discursive pyramid underneath it. See her other important discussions of AIDS from a theoretical perspective that combines Foucauldian theory, feminist theories, and linguistics in Treichler (1987, 1988, 1989a, 1989b, 1991, 1992b, 1993).

## I. Paralysis or Breakthrough

1. See Kramer's essay "The FDA's Callous Response to AIDS" (1989, pp. 140-44) for a discussion of a battery of potentially useful and less toxic drugs than AZT that in Kramer's view have not received sufficient attention by the FDA.

2. For an activist description and analysis of the alternative treatment movement, see ACT UP (1990b).

3. The Orphan Drug Act, signed on January 4, 1983, and sponsored by Representative Henry Waxman and Senator Orrin Hatch, encouraged the development and manufacture of drugs that treat diseases affecting so few people that the cost of developing the drug far outweighs potential profits. The drug company may claim up to 63 percent of the cost of clinical studies as a tax credit. Most important, the company is granted an exclusive license to market the drug for up to seven years.

4. The Treatment IND Amendment, formalized in May 1987 by the FDA, allows drugs still in the investigation stages (there are normally three stages in the clinical study) to be used by persons with serious or life-threatening illnesses for which there is no other treatment. The idea, however, sounds better than the reality. See ACT UP (1988, pp. 13-14, 20-23) for a critique of the amendment and a description of its drastic failure in the pentamidine case.

5. Descriptions of scientific discovery in AIDS often employ the language of "masquerade"; other AIDS drugs being developed have been narrated in this way. For instance, CD4 is a substance that resembles a binding site on the human cell that attracts HIV. When HIV binds with free-floating, synthetic CD4, a toxin is released to destroy HIV. The metaphoric descriptions of CD4 include "synthetic copies," "false targets," "a guided missile," "a poison-carrying missile," "new biological weapon," and "false handle to which the virus clings." Descriptions of its action include "decoy," "lure," "mop up," "flood," "hijack," and "painting poison on a homing molecule" (see Chase, 1988b, 1988c, 1988d). Other interesting nomenclatures are "disinfectants" (e.g., Immunozone treatment), appetite-stimulating drugs to counter weight loss (e.g., Megace), blood filtration outside the body (e.g., Prosorba immunoabsorption device), "modified poisons" to select and kill HIV (e.g., pseudomonas exotoxin A), "anti-sense drugs" to block the production of new viral material, and "blood warming."

6. Strategic reasons supported the shift from a focus on AIDS specifically to a focus on health-care issues. AIDS activists and advocate groups contended that the shift would broaden the funding base for AIDS research. The move was strategically important despite its contribution to the normalization of AIDS and the failure to change the narrow focus of HIV-based research.

7. Randomized, double-blinded, and placebo-controlled drug trials are the standard methodology employed by medical researchers to test the effectiveness of drugs. Test

subjects are randomly put into two groups, one of which receives the experimental drug and the other a placebo (an inert substance). Neither the subjects nor the researchers know which the subjects are taking until the trials are complete.

8. The "endpoint" of a clinical trial refers to the hallmark by which the effectiveness of an experimental drug is measured. For a long time, the FDA required that drugs for HIV infection be proven to extend life or to slow the progression of AIDS, endpoints that can take many years to establish because of the slow progress of the disease. Endpoints therefore have a profound effect on how fast drugs can be approved. On February 14, 1991, the FDA overturned its previous position and accepted the use of the CD4 helper cell test as a measure of an antiviral drug's effectiveness. For a description and an analysis of this change, see Project Inform (1991).

9. For discussions of the problems of the *Native*'s various positions on AIDS, see Crimp (1987) and Kinsella (1989).

10. To compare the *Native* roundtable with another discussion where a diversity of opinions and experiences of AZT was expressed, see "The Pros and Cons of Taking AZT: A Roundtable Discussion," 1988. See also Schick (1989b).

11. Class and gender differences constitute major factors in determining whether one is likely to be able to participate in the clinical trials, whether one can afford expensive drugs like AZT without being in a trial, or for that matter whether one is likely to be a participant in the activist movement so as to be informed and active in the struggle for treatment.

## 2. Articulating the (Im)possible

1. See Erni (1992a) for a theoretical discussion of the relations between the material body and cultural representations in the context of the AIDS crisis. Other useful work on the subject can be found in Gallop (1988); Levin and Solomon (1990); and Scarry (1985).

2. Examples of media descriptions of HIV can be found in Barber (1985); Brownlee (1990); Chase (1988d); Kolata (1988a; 1988b; 1988c; 1988e); Schmeck (1988); and Seligman (1988).

3. For a discussion of a video critique of the representation of PWA Kenny Ramsaur, see Gever (1987). For a discussion of Fabian Bridges's story, see Crimp (1992).

4. See Dawidoff (1989) and Ruskin (1988).

5. Religious connotations of the image are abundantly present in the photograph. The basic iconographic reference lies in the hands of a divine figure (perhaps Christ) in the portrait on the wall in the background, the hand of a priest extended from the space off-frame, and the sheltering hands of the parents.

6. Some sample stories of PWAs as victimizers covered in the *New York Times* in 1987 include:

• March, Milwaukee: A woman journalist discussed the anger and despair she felt because her husband was bisexual and dying of AIDS. She feared that her children had been infected.

• April, Arizona: Adrian Morris of the U.S. Army was charged with aggravated assault for having sexual relations with two other soldiers, a man and a woman. A court martial was expected.

• June, Los Angeles: Murder charges were filed against a mentally ill gay man who twice sold his alleged "AIDS-infected blood" to the Plasma Production Associates.

• October, Suffolk County, N.Y.: Police were trying to locate any other "victims" of Michael Hawkrigg, who was HIV-positive and was charged with sodomizing a sixteen-year-old boy.

7. In clinical trials, science demands controlled and idealized subjects for experimentation; the "pure body" is dogmatically required as the experimental subject. Scientists often attempt to maintain a rigorous surveillance of the participants' use of the experimental drugs, which means banning their use of any other substances during the trial period. As a scientific standard, this may not be an unreasonable request. But as a reality, such a "clean" population does not exist. Many patients involved in the trials frequently admit that they do not reveal all their clinical experience of symptoms to the researchers, nor do they reveal that they have been using other experimental treatments while participating in trials. As ACT UP founder Larry Kramer reports, "There is no way the FDA, or anyone else, can set up genuinely 'controlled' studies. Such studies require people to certify that they have or have not suffered from certain diseases in the past. But people with AIDS will say or do anything to obtain a drug or join a test. They forge their medical records, and, because the FDA bureaucracy is so entrenched, every doctor I know lies for them" (1989, p. 142). The scientific protocol that demands "clean bodies" to be tested is thus illusory. The insistence on adhering to an idealistic trial method reveals science's fantasy for unblemished drugs and pure bodies.

8. See Gevitz (1988) for a discussion of the history of alternative medicine in the United States.

9. At the same conference, which has been lauded as a forum for "comprehensive" viewpoints, the symposium on alternative medicine was underpublicized. Many papers on alternative treatments for AIDS were not accepted (ACT UP, 1990b). Fewer than four hundred people attended the Advanced Immune Discoveries Symposium held by Dr. Laurance Badgley (Russell, 1990).

10. In the report, ACT UP (1990b) demands the following changes: (1) NIH and private medical research centers must stop boycotting research on alternative AIDS treatments; (2) Medicaid, Medicare, and private health insurance policies must end their exclusions of alternative practitioners and treatments; (3) all states must establish licensing for the alternative health professions; (4) state law enforcement agencies must stop the arbitrary enforcement of medical licensing laws against physicians using alternative approaches; (5) government and private health organizations must stop waging propaganda campaigns against alternative health care in the name of "fighting quackery"; (6) public hospitals and clinics must provide at least minimal alternative treatment services, particularly in poor communities; (7) medical institutions must offer referrals to alternative treatment resources; (8) AIDS conferences, directories, newsletters, and training programs must stop excluding alternative practitioners and treatments; and (9) medical institutions and government health agencies must seek input from the alternative AIDS treatment community.

11. The uneasiness experienced by users of alternative medicine is part of the wider problem of PWAs' relation to medicine. Whatever challenge alternative treatment may pose to official medicine, it represents a contradiction for PWAs: they recognize the ideology of organized scientific undertakings, but they depend on biomedical research to develop the possible cure for AIDS because social and economic resources remain there. This contradiction is particularly problematic for the gay communities (see Bayer, 1985). To challenge biomedical authority is to recognize at the same time the uneasy reality of its potential contribution.

## 3. Temporality and the Politics of AIDS Science

1. I am aware of the argument, particularly in postmodern criticisms, that rightly suggests that time has been a dominant category of analysis in critical social theory, and that

time has subordinated a consideration of space. I do not intend to resubmerge space in favor of time; my aim is to supplement, not substitute. I want to make the strongest possible case for the hypothesis that AIDS research is more strongly anchored in a politics of time than in a politics of space.

2. Scientists who advocated the "dormancy theory," for example, argued that after infection HIV remained largely inactive followed by a sudden burst of infective activities at a later time. Their view thus placed more emphasis on variations of factors beyond HIV infection in determining the patient's course of illness.

3. For a brief discussion of the Tuskegee Syphilis Study, see Treichler (1991). See also ACT UP (1988) and Breo (1988) for brief descriptions of the Elixir Sulfanilamide and Thalidomide incidents. Breo argues that these events were key markers in the evolution of the regulatory health polity represented by the FDA.

4. This has been seen in, among other things, the emergence of the teaching of scientific method in medical schools, transforming medical education into a way of learning scientific matters involving public health and increasing specialization of physicians as researchers.

5. For discussions of other important problems of the clinical trials process, such as the debates over informed consent, the use of placebos, and the biased selection of research subjects, which are not directly related to the question of timing, see Kramer (1989) and ACT UP (1988).

6. The specific criteria are as follows: (1) the drug is intended to treat a serious or immediately life-threatening disease; (2) no comparable or satisfactory alternative or other therapy exists to treat that stage of the disease in the intended population; (3) the drug is under investigation in a controlled clinical trial under an IND in effect for the trial, or all clinical trials have been completed; and (4) the sponsor for the controlled clinical trial is actively pursuing marketing approval of the investigational drug with due diligence (F. Young, 1988, p. 2268).

7. In this argument, my intent is not to favor one kind of experimentation over another, or to favor abolishing clinical trials once and for all. I seek to disentangle some of the structural conditions of a certain practice in an underlying, broad context within which some ideas about the "social contract" (with all its ethical implications) are preferred and perpetuated, while others are not properly honored. It seems that the subject's wish to negotiate the space and time of treatment and experimentation, either individually or collectively, is often received with suspicion and skepticism or is sometimes ignored entirely.

8. See ACT UP (1990a); Arno and Feiden (1992); Nussbaum (1990); and Schick (1989a).

9. Nowhere is the exertion of power to the body based on a rational language of temporality more forceful than in the medical discourse of the female body. Historically, the female body has often been the site of medicine's temporal control. The most prominent example is the biomedical discourse of childbirth. For example, Emily Martin (1987) analyzes the obstetrical literature on "labor" and discovers that the image of the uterus during labor often parallels that of the factory worker in time and motion studies. The manner in which the uterus acts during labor is expressed in terms familiar to any student of time and motion studies as those used to analyze and control the worker's body movements. Deviation from the set rates of labor is therefore perceived as the body's disorder. According to Martin, some medical texts go so far as to suggest that labor contractions are correlated to the woman's emotional state, despite evidence that uterine contractions are involuntary. Thus, cultural assumptions fold onto one another, defining the woman's body first as a machine, then casting suspicion over its efficiency, which therefore gives way to the legiti-

macy of administering drugs that would control the rate of dilation and contraction, an external manipulation to assure maximum productivity.

The temporal control of the female body in medicine also pervades the field of therapy and treatment. See Bassuk (1986) for an analysis of one of the best-known treatments offered to women in the late nineteenth century—the rest cure. The examples of childbirth and the rest cure suggest that it is possible not only to hold an empirically based discourse about an individual (constructed around the uterus's rate of contraction and the nervous system's adaptation to the pace of life), but also to ask the body to act, to perform, to produce.

10. Such a redesign of the body also requires a spatial organization; in fact the Taylorist labor process received its enduring authority from the photographic images detailing the worker's body in motion. Also, the Taylorist mode of control has undergone change. The rise of Fordism and neo-Fordism in the 1960s promoted a different relation between the rhythm of labor and the rhythm of production. In essence, with the advent of machine tools, cybernetics, and assembly lines in industrial settings (most notably the car-manufacturing industry), the rhythm of labor and the rhythm of production have been made completely independent of one another. For a general discussion of such transformations, see Alliez and Feher (1987).

## 4. Power and Ambivalence

1. Minkowitz has asked, "As the group [ACT UP] grows in size and power, a debate is raging: Should ACT UP be an AIDS lobby, a Gay Liberation front, a New Left collective, or all of the above?" (1990, pp. 19-20). For reference to the internal division of the activist group that eventually led to a split of ACT UP/San Francisco, see Pepper (1990); Shilts (1989a); and Vollmer (1990).

2. Generally speaking, the media's depiction of expressions of dissent (direct action, protest, strikes, and so on) always implies violence. As John Hartley has argued: "Manifestations of dissent are seen as containing the 'threat of violence,' and the threat of violence is 'anti-social' in the profoundest sense. Exactly *whose* 'society' is being so threatened is not an open question, since the consensual model requires 'society' to be everyone. Dissidents, then, are mad or malicious" (1982, p. 84).

3. For a general consideration of the questions of civil disobedience and militancy and their relation to ACT UP and other activist groups, see Cohen (1989). For a defense of ACT UP's philosophy, see Novick (1989).

4. These descriptions of ACT UP are found in Barinaga (1990); Crossen (1989); DeParle (1990); Gross (1990b); Kolata, (1990b); Leo, (1990); Salholz et al. (1988, 1990); Shilts (1989b, 1989c); and Spiers (1989).

## 5. An Epistemology of Curing.

1. These findings are compiled from the following sources: Albert (1986a, 1986b); Altman (1986); Baker (1986); Colby and Cook (1991); Dearing and Rogers (1988); Karpf (1988); Kinsella (1989); McAllister (1990); Patton (1990); and Treichler (1987).

2. The crucial difference is that the theory of encoding/decoding is based on a communication or transactional model of analysis, and the theory of articulation is based on a contextual and structural model of analysis. The transactional model of analysis emphasizes the distinctive moments and instances in the (significatory) play of cultural relations. A contextual model of analysis emphasizes relations and formations within the totality of culture. Encoding/decoding lacks the dialecticism of the theory of articulation.

3. The language of purification is most evident in the discussion of GLQ223, also

known as trichosanthin and most commonly referred to as Compound Q. Briefly, Compound Q appears to selectively kill infected T-cells and macrophages, the common types of immune system cells to which the HIV binds. The drug appears to kill these infected cells while doing little damage to healthy cells. In vitro tests have proved it to be more potent and more selective than any other known anti-HIV compound; the discovery came through the work of Dr. Michael McGrath. In 1989, news of it electrified the AIDS communities. But Project Inform (1989) reveals that word of McGrath's findings had leaked out as early as 1987, when an official blackout was imposed, hiding from public view the fact that laboratory research of Compound Q was going on, as FDA forms were filed and patent rights sought. For discussions of Compound Q by the press, see Goldstein and Massa (1989); Kingston (1989); Kolata (1989b); and Perlman (1990).

4. See Latour and Woolgar (1986) and Poovey (1991) for the argument that scientific or historical discourses cannot readily be separated from fictional ones. Also, see Miller (1990) for a recent account of new developments in narrative theories and of their relevance to cultural struggles.

# Bibliography

ACT UP. (1988, September 21). *FDA Action Handbook*. Manuscript.

ACT UP. (1990a, May 1). *A Critique of AIDS Clinical Trials Group*. Manuscript by Treatment and Data Committee.

ACT UP. (1990b, June). Alternative and holistic AIDS treatments. Press release during the Sixth International Conference on AIDS, San Francisco.

AIDS and 1962. (1988, July 14). *Wall Street Journal*, p. 26.

Albert, E. (1986a). Acquired immune deficiency syndrome: The victim and the press. *Studies in Communication*, 3, 135-158.

Albert, E. (1986b). Illness and deviance: The response of the press to AIDS. In D. A. Feldman and T. M. Johnson (Eds.), *The Social Dimensions of AIDS: Method and Theory*. New York: Praeger. 163-178.

Alliez, E., and M. Feher. (1987). The luster of capital. *Zone*, 1/2, 315-359.

Altman, D. (1986). *AIDS in the Mind of America*. Garden City, N.Y.: Anchor.

Amara, R. (1988, November/December). Health care tomorrow. *Futurist*, 16-20.

Annas, G. (1990). Faith (healing), hope, and charity at the FDA: The politics of AIDS drug trials. In L. Gostin (Ed.), *AIDS and the Health Care System*. New Haven: Yale University Press. 183-194.

Arno, P. S., and K. L. Feiden. (1992). *Against the Odds: The Story of AIDS Drug Development, Politics & Profits*. New York: HarperCollins.

Arras, J. (1990, September/October). Non-compliance in AIDS research. *Hastings Center Report*, pp. 24-32.

Baker, A. J. (1986). The portrayal of AIDS in the media: An analysis of articles in the *New York Times*. In D. A. Feldman and T. M. Johnson (Eds.), *The Social Dimensions of AIDS: Method and Theory*. New York: Praeger. 179-194.

Barber, J., et al. (1985, August 12). The indiscriminate killer. *Maclean*, p. 38.

Barinaga, M. (1990, June 8). AIDS conference: science or circus? *Science*, p. 1181.

Barthes, R. (1988). Semiology and medicine. In R. Barthes, *The Semiotic Challenge*. New York: Hill and Wang. 202-213.

Bassuk, E. (1986). The rest cure: Repetition or resolution of Victorian women's conflicts? In S. Suleiman (Ed.), *The Female Body in Western Culture*. Cambridge: Harvard University Press. 139-151.

Bayer, R. (1985, Autumn). AIDS and the gay community: Between the specter and the promise of medicine. *Social Research*, 52(3), 581-606.

Boffey, P. (1988a, April 30). Official blames shortage of staff for delay in testing AIDS drugs. *New York Times*, pp. A1+.

Boffey, P. (1988b, July 5). New initiatives to speed AIDS drugs is assailed. *New York Times*. p. C1.

Boffey, P. (1988c, July 24). Tests of potential drug for AIDS beginning after months of delay. *New York Times*, p. A19.

Boffey, P. (1988d, July 24). FDA will allow AIDS patients to import AIDS medicines. *New York Times*, p. A1.

Boffey, P. (1988e, August 7). U.S. studies ways to speed drugs for seriously ill. *New York Times*, p. A1.

Boffey, P. (1988f, July 14). FDA is pessimistic on drugs to fight AIDS. *New York Times*, p. B9.

Boffin, T. and S. Gupta (Eds.). (1990). *Ecstatic Antibodies: Resisting the AIDS Mythology*. London: Rivers Oram.

Brand, D. (1987, June 1). "It was too good to be true": Faking data: A mental-retardation researcher faces grim charges. *Time*, p. 59.

Brandt, A. (1987). *No Magic Bullet: A Social History of Venereal Disease in the United States since 1880*. New York: Oxford University Press.

Breo, D. (1988, September 25). Where are the drugs to cure AIDS? *Chicago Tribune Magazine*, pp. 11-37.

Brownlee, S. (1990, July 2). The body at war: Baring the secrets of the immune system. *U.S. News & World Report*, pp. 48-54.

Burroughs Wellcome. (1990, June). *The age of antivirals: A new era in medicine*. Press release during the Sixth International Conference on AIDS, San Francisco.

Buxton, R. (1991, Spring). "After it happened . . .": The battle to present AIDS in television drama. *Velvet Light Trap*, 27, 37-48.

Callen, M. (1990). *Surviving AIDS*. New York: HarperCollins.

Cannon, W. B. (1945). *The Way of an Investigator*. New York: Hafner.

Carey, J. (1990, November 5). NIH is not the institution it was: Funding cuts, scandals, and politics are taking toll on the venerable biomedical research agency. *Business Week*, pp. 145-148.

Carpenter, B. (1989, May 8). The body's master controls. *U.S. News & World Report*, pp. 57-59.

Carter, E., and S. Watney (Eds.). (1989). *Taking Liberties: AIDS and Cultural Politics*. London: Serpent's Tail.

Chase, M. (1988a, April 28). Defusing a bomb: Doctors and patients hope AZT will help to stave off AIDS. *Wall Street Journal*, p. 1.

Chase, M. (1988b, June 3). Group enters field studying CD4 for AIDS. *Wall Street Journal*, p. 22.

Chase, M. (1988c, June 15). Harvard researcher sees poor chances of success for a popular AIDS therapy. *Wall Street Journal*, p. 28.

Chase, M. (1988d, August 4). AIDS virus in infected people mutates at a dizzying rate, two studies show. *Wall Street Journal*, p. 24.

Chase, M. (1988e, August 10). Human tests are set to begin today on new drug therapy to fight AIDS. *Wall Street Journal*, p. 24.

Chase, M. (1989, March 3). Homing in: Science edges closer to designing drugs to defeat AIDS virus. *Wall Street Journal*, pp. A1, A5.

Clark, J., et al. (1975). Subcultures, cultures, and class: A theoretical overview. *Working Papers in Cultural Studies*, 7/8.

Clark, M., et al. (1985, August 5). AIDS exiles in Paris. *Newsweek*, p. 71.

Cohen, C. (1989, November/December). Militant morality: civil disobedience and bioethics. *Hastings Center Report*, pp. 23-25.

Colby, D., and T. Cook. (1991, Summer). Epidemics and agendas: The politics of nightly news coverage of AIDS. *Journal of Health Politics, Policy, and Law*, 16(2), 215-249.

Colby, D., and T. Cook. (1992). The mass-mediated epidemic: The politics of AIDS on the nightly network news. In E. Fee and D. M. Fox (Eds.), *AIDS: The Making of a Chronic Disease*. Berkeley and Los Angeles: University of California Press. 84-124.

Comroe, J. (1977). *Retrospectroscope: Insights into Medical Discovery*. Menlo Park, Calif.: Von Gehr.

Coulter, H. (1987). *AIDS and Syphilis: The Hidden Link*. Berkeley: North Atlantic.

Cowley, G., et al. (1990, June 25). AIDS: The next ten years. *Newsweek*, pp. 20-27.

Crewdson, J. (1989, November 19). The great AIDS quest. *Chicago Tribune*, pp. E1-E16.

Crimp, D. (1987, Winter). How to have promiscuity in an epidemic. *October*, 43, 237-271.

Crimp, D. (1989, Winter). Mourning and militancy. *October*, 51, 3-18.

Crimp, D. (1992). Portraits of people with AIDS. In L. Grossberg, C. Nelson, and P. Treichler (Eds.), *Cultural Studies*. New York: Routledge. 117-133.

Crimp, D. (Ed.). (1987, Winter). AIDS: Cultural analysis/cultural activism [special issue]. *October, 43*.

Crimp, D., and A. Rolston. (1990). *AIDS Demo Graphics*. Seattle: Bay Press.

Crossen, C. (1989, December 7). Shock troops: AIDS activist group harasses and provokes to make its point. *Wall Street Journal*, p. A1.

Dale, H. H. (1948). Accident and opportunism in medical research. *British Medical Journal, 2*, 451-455.

Davis, J. (1989). *Defending the Body: Unraveling the Mysteries of Immunology*. New York: Atheneum.

Dawidoff, R. (1989). The NAMES Project. In J. Preston (Ed.), *Personal Dispatches: Writers Confront AIDS*. New York: St. Martin's. 145-151.

Dearing, J. W., and E. M. Rogers. (1988, May). *The agenda-setting process for the issue of AIDS*. Paper presented at the International Communication Association Conference, New Orleans.

Deciphering the system: An interview with Jay Lipner. (1991, January/February). *PWA Coalition Newsline*, pp. 18-22.

DeParle, J. (1990, January 3). Rude, rash, effective, ACT UP shifts AIDS policy. *New York Times*, p. B1.

Duesberg, P. (1988, July 29). HIV is not the cause of AIDS. *Science, 241*, 514-517.

Dying for dollars [editorial]. (1990, December 17). *New Republic*, pp. 7-8.

Edelman, L. (1989, Winter). The plague of discourse: Politics, literary theory, and AIDS. *South Atlantic Quarterly, 88*(1), 301-317.

Edelman, L. (1993). The mirror and the tank: "AIDS," subjectivity, and the rhetoric of activism. In T. Murphy and S. Poirier (Eds.), *Writing AIDS: Gay Literature, Language, and Analysis*. New York: Columbia University Press. 9-38.

Edgar, H., and D. Rothman. (1991). New rules for new drugs: The challenge of AIDS to the regulatory process. In D. Nelkin, D. Willis, and S. Parris (Eds.), *A Disease of Society: Cultural and Institutional Responses to AIDS*. Cambridge: Cambridge University Press. 84-115.

Edgar, H., and D. Rothman. (1992). Scientific rigor and medical realities: Placebo trials in cancer and AIDS research. In E. Fee and D. M. Fox (Eds.), *AIDS: The Making of a Chronic Disease*. Berkeley and Los Angeles: University of California Press. 194-206.

Eisenberg (1986, April). *Private trust/public confidence in science and medicine: The genesis of fear*. Paper presented at the annual meeting of the American Society of Law and Medicine, Boston.

Enthoven, A. (1989, July 13). A "cost-unconscious" medical system. *New York Times*, p. A19.

Epstein, S. (1991, April/June). Democratic science? AIDS activism and the contested construction of knowledge. *Socialist Review, 21*, 35-64.

Erni, J. (1992a). Intensive care: Mapping the body-politics of AIDS. *Praxis, 3*, 47-69.

Erni, J. (1992b). Articulating the (im)possible: Popular media and the cultural politics of "curing AIDS." *Communication, 13*, 39-56.

Farber, C. (1989, November). Sins of omission. *Spin*.

Finkelstein, J. L. (1990, July/August). Biomedicine and technocratic power. *Hastings Center Report*, pp. 13-16.

Foucault, M. (1975). *The Birth of the Clinic: An Archaeology of Medical Perception* (A. M. Sheridan Smith, Trans.). New York: Vintage.

Foucault, M. (1980). Two lectures. In C. Gordon (Ed.), *Power/Knowledge: Selected Interviews and Other Writings, 1972-1977*. New York: Pantheon. 78-108.

Foucault, M. (1981, Spring). Questions of method: An interview with Michel Foucault. *Ideology and Consciousness*, 8, 3-14.

Foucault, M. (1984). Right of death and power over life. In P. Rabinow (Ed.), *The Foucault Reader*. New York: Pantheon. 258-272.

Fox, D. (1988). AIDS and the American health polity: The history and prospects of a crisis of authority. In E. Fox and D. Fox (Eds.), *AIDS: The Burdens of History*. Berkeley and Los Angeles: University of California Press. 316-343.

Fox, D. (1990a, Summer). Chronic disease and disadvantage: The new politics of HIV infection. *Journal of Health Politics, Policy and Law*, 15(2), 341-355.

Fox, D. (1990b, Fall). Health policy and the politics of research in the United States. *Journal of Health Politics, Policy and Law*, 15(3), 481-499.

Fox, D. M. (1992). The politics of HIV infection: 1989-1990 as years of change. In E. Fee and D. M. Fox (Eds.), *AIDS: The Making of a Chronic Disease*. Berkeley and Los Angeles: University of California Press. 125-143.

Freund, P. (1982). Holistic medicine and re-claiming the body. In P. Freund, *The Civilized Body: Social Domination, Control, and Health*. Philadelphia: Temple University Press. 27-38.

Fuss, D. (Ed.). (1991). *Inside/Out: Lesbian Theories, Gay Theories*. New York: Routledge.

Gallop, G. (1988). *Thinking through the Body*. New York: Columbia University Press.

Geitner, P. (1988, June 19). Desperation drives victims to try unapproved drugs. *Champaign-Urbana News-Gazette*, p. B4.

Gever, M. (1987, Winter). Pictures of sickness: Stuart Marshall's *Bright Eyes*. *October*, 43, 109-126.

Gevitz, N. (Ed.). (1988). *Other Healers: Unorthodox Medicine in America*. Baltimore: Johns Hopkins University Press.

Gilman, S. (1988). *Disease and Representation: Images of Illness from Madness to AIDS*. Ithaca: Cornell University Press.

Goldstein, R. (1989, March 14). Bishop Berkeley's virus: The two cultures of AIDS. *Village Voice*, pp. 49-51.

Goldstein, R. (1991). The implicated and the immune: Responses to AIDS in the arts and popular culture. In D. Nelkin, D. Willis, and S. Parris (Eds.), *A Disease of Society: Cultural and Institutional Responses to AIDS*. Cambridge: Cambridge University Press. 17-42.

Goldstein, R., and R. Massa. (1989, May 30). Compound Q: Hope and hype. *Village Voice*, pp. 29-34.

Graham, M. (1991, January). The quiet drug revolution. *Atlantic*, pp. 34-40.

Gross, J. (1990a, June 21). Protest, not poignancy, marks AIDS gathering. *New York Times*, p. B5.

Gross, J. (1990b, June 24). City hears harmony, with a few jarring notes. *New York Times*, p. A23.

Grossberg, L. (1986, Summer). On postmodernism and articulation: An interview with Stuart Hall. *Journal of Communication Inquiry*, 10(2), pp. 45-60.

Grossberg, L. (1990). The formation of cultural studies: An American in Birmingham. *Strategies*, 2, 114-149.

Grover, J. Z. (1989, Summer). Visible lesions: Images of people with AIDS. *Afterimage*, 17(1), 10-16.

Grover, J. Z. (1992). AIDS, keywords, and cultural work. In L. Grossberg, C. Nelson, and P. Treichler (Eds.), *Cultural Studies*. New York: Routledge. 227-239.

Hall, S. (1985, June). Signification, representation, ideology: Althusser and the post-structuralist debates. *Critical Studies in Mass Communication, 2*(2), 91-114.

Hall, S. (1992). Cultural studies and its theoretical legacies. In L. Grossberg, C. Nelson, and P. Treichler (Eds.), *Cultural Studies.* New York: Routledge. 277-294.

Hall, S., et al. (1978). *Policing the Crisis: Mugging, the State, and Law and Order.* New York: Holmes & Meier.

Hammer, J. (1988, August 15). Inside the illegal AIDS drug trade. *Newsweek,* pp. 41-42.

Haraway, D. (1989). The bio-politics of postmodern bodies: Determinations of self in immune system discourse. *Differences, 1*(1), 3-43.

Haraway, D. (1992). The promises of monsters: A regenerative politics for inappropriate/d others. In L. Grossberg, C. Nelson, and P. Treichler (Eds.), *Cultural Studies.* New York: Routledge. 295-337.

Harrington, M. (1990, March 13). Anatomy of a disaster: Why is federal AIDS research at a standstill? *Village Voice,* pp. 40-41.

Hartley, J. (1982). *Understanding News.* New York: Methuen.

Haseltine, W., and F. Wong-Staal. (1988, October). The molecular biology of the AIDS virus. *Scientific American, 259*(4), 52-63.

Horton, M. (1989). Bugs, drugs, and placebos: The opulence of truth, or how to make a treatment decision in an epidemic. In E. Carter and S. Watney (Eds.), *Taking Liberties: AIDS and Cultural Politics.* London: Serpent's Tail. 161-182.

Jaroff, L. (1990, September 24). Giant step for gene therapy. *Time,* pp. 74-76.

Jaroff, L. (1991, August 26). Crisis in the labs. *Time,* pp. 45-51.

Juhasz, A. (1992). From within: Alternative AIDS media by women. *Praxis, 3,* 23-45.

Karpf, A. (1988). *Doctoring the Media: The Reporting of Health and Medicine.* New York: Routledge, Chapman and Hall.

Kingston, T. (1989, May). Q: The politics of hope vs. the business of AIDS. *Bay Times,* pp. 5-6.

Kinsella, J. (1989). *Covering the Plague: AIDS and the American Media.* New Brunswick, N.J.: Rutgers University Press.

Klusacek, A., and K. Morrison. (Eds.). (1992). *A Leap in the Dark: AIDS, Art and Contemporary Cultures.* Montreal: Vehicule.

Kolata, G. (1988a, March 22). Fatal strategy of AIDS virus grows clearer. *New York Times,* p. C1.

Kolata, G. (1988b, June 5). AIDS virus found to hide in cells, eluding detection by normal tests. *New York Times,* p. A1.

Kolata, G. (1988c, June 7). The evolving biology of AIDS: Scavenger cell looms large. *New York Times,* p. C1.

Kolata, G. (1988d, July 10). AIDS patients and their above-ground underground. *New York Times,* p. E32.

Kolata, G. (1988e, November 15). Researchers discover how AIDS virus lurks in bone marrow cells. *New York Times,* p. C3.

Kolata, G. (1988f, November 26). Odd alliance would speed new drugs. *New York Times,* p. A9.

Kolata, G. (1988g, December 18). Recruiting problems in New York slowing U.S. trials of AIDS drug. *New York Times,* p. A1.

Kolata, G. (1989a, June 26). AIDS studies head seeks wide access to drugs in tests. *New York Times,* p. A1.

Kolata, G. (1989b, September 19). Critics fault secret effort to test AIDS drug. *New York Times,* p. C1.

Kolata, G. (1990a, March 26). Radical change urged in testing of AIDS drugs. *New York Times*, p. A1.

Kolata, G. (1990b, March 11). Advocates' tactics on AIDS issues provoking warnings of a backlash. *New York Times*, p. D5.

Kopkind, A. (1993, May 3). The gay moment. *Nation*, pp. 577, 590-602.

Kramer, L. (1989). *Reports from the Holocaust: The Making of an AIDS Activist*. New York: St. Martin's.

Kupelian, D., et al. (1990, March). The battle over AIDS: Disease control vs. hysteria control. *New Dimension*, pp. 20-25.

Laclau, E., and C. Mouffe. (1985). *Hegemony and Socialist Strategy*. London: Verso.

Landers, T. (1988, January/February). Bodies and antibodies: A crisis in representation. *Independent*, 11(1), 18-24.

Latour, B., and S. Woolgar. (1986). *Laboratory Life: The Construction of Scientific Facts*. Princeton: Princeton University Press.

Lauritsen, J. (1989a, January 2). On the AZT front: Part I. *New York Native*.

Lauritsen, J. (1989b, January 16). On the AZT front: Part II. *New York Native*.

Lauritsen, J. (1989c, September). The case against AZT. *PWA Coalition Newsline*, 56-58.

Lauritsen, J. (1990, March 19). A "state-of-the-art" AZT conference. *New York Native*, pp. 17-20.

Lederberg, J. (1988). Medical science, infectious disease, and the unity of humankind. *Journal of American Medical Association*, 260(5), 684-685.

Leibowitch, J. (1985). *A Strange Virus of Unknown Origin* (R. Howard, Trans.). New York: Ballantine.

Leo, J. (1990, February 5). When activism becomes gangsterism. *U.S. News & World Report*, p. 18.

Lerner, S. (1991, May). Women . . . AIDS . . . and the media. *PWA Coalition Newsline*, pp. 23-45.

Levin, D., and G. Solomon. (1990). The discursive formation of the body in the history of medicine. *Journal of Medicine and Philosophy*, 15, 515-537.

Maccani, J. (1990, November 19). Maccani responds to Lauritsen. *GLC Voice* (Minneapolis), p. 7.

Marshall, S. (1990). Picturing deviancy. In T. Boffin and S. Gupta (Eds.), *Ecstatic Antibodies: Resisting the AIDS Mythology*. London: Rivers Oram. 19-36.

Martin, E. (1987). *The Woman in the Body*. Boston: Beacon.

Marwick, C. (1988, August 12). Philosophy on trial: Examining ethics of clinical investigations. *Journal of the American Medical Association*, 260(6), 749-751.

Masters, R. (1990, March). AIDS and denial. *New Dimension*, pp. 44-49.

McAllister, M. (1990). *Medicalization in the news media: A comparison of AIDS coverage in three newspapers*. Unpublished doctoral dissertation, University of Illinois at Urbana-Champaign.

McGrath, R. (1990). Dangerous liaison: Health, disease, and representation. In T. Boffin and S. Gupta (Eds.), *Ecstatic Antibodies: Resisting the AIDS Mythology*. London: Rivers Oram. 142-155.

Metz, C. (1990). Photography and fetish. In C. Squiers (Ed.), *The Critical Image: Essays on Contemporary Photography*. Seattle: Bay Press. 155-164.

Miller, J. H. (1990). Narrative. In F. Lentricchia and T. McLaughlin (Eds.), *Critical Terms for Literary Study*. Chicago: University of Chicago Press. 66-79.

Miller, J. (Ed.). (1992). *Fluid Exchanges: Artists and Critics in the AIDS Crisis*. Toronto: University of Toronto Press.

Minkowitz, D. (1990, June 5). ACT UP at a crossroads. *Village Voice*, pp. 19-22.

Monmaney, T., et al. (1987, June 1). Preying on AIDS patients. *Newsweek*, pp. 52-54.

Murphy, T. (1991, March/April). No time for an AIDS backlash. *Hastings Center Report*, pp. 7-11.

Murphy, T., and S. Poirier. (Eds.). (1993). *Writing AIDS: Gay Literature, Language, and Analysis*. New York: Columbia University Press.

Myers, G. (1990). Making a discovery: Narratives of split genes. In C. Nash (Ed.), *Narrative in Culture: The Uses of Storytelling in the Sciences, Philosophy, and Literature*. New York: Routledge. 102-126.

Myers, M., and J. La Montagnier. (1987). Clinical trials of drugs for the treatment of AIDS. *AMA Information on AIDS for the Practicing Physician*, *3*, 5-8.

Nash, C. (1990). *Narrative in Culture: The Uses of Storytelling in the Sciences, Philosophy, and Literature*. New York: Routledge.

Nation's public health system is in disarray, major report finds. (1988, October/November). *Nation's Health*, p. 1+.

Native roundtable: Concentration without walls. (1989, December 18). *New York Native*, pp. 17-20.

New ideas for new drugs. (1988, December 28). *Wall Street Journal*, p. A6.

Nickles, T. (1985). Beyond divorce: Current status of the discovery debate. *Philosophy of Science*, *52*, 177-206.

Nightingale, S. (1989). *The role of the FDA in the AIDS drug development process*. Paper presented at the American Association for the Advancement of Science Symposium on Clinical Trials of AIDS Drugs: Issues of Science, Ethics, and Confidentiality, San Francisco.

Novick, A. (1989, November/December). Civil disobedience in time of AIDS. *Hastings Center Report*, pp. 35-36.

Nunokawa, J. (1991). "All the sad young men": AIDS and the work of mourning. In D. Fuss (Ed.), *Inside/Out: Lesbian Theories, Gay Theories*. New York: Routledge. 311-323.

Nussbaum, B. (1990). *Good Intentions: How Big Business and the Medical Establishment Are Corrupting the Fight against AIDS*. New York: Atlantic Monthly Press.

O'Reilly, B. (1990, November 5). The inside story of the AIDS drug. *Fortune*, pp. 112-129.

Panem, S. (1988). *The AIDS Bureaucracy*. Cambridge: Harvard University Press.

Patton, C. (1990). *Inventing AIDS*. New York: Routledge.

Pepper, R. (1990, October 10). Schism slices ACT UP in two: San Francisco chapter splits in debate over focus. *Outweek*, pp. 12-14.

Perlman, D. (1990, June 23). S. F. group reports on Compound Q. *San Francisco Chronicle*, p. A11.

Poovey, M. (1991). Review of Bruce Clark and Wendell Aycock's *The Body and the Text: Comparative Essays in Literature and Medicine*. *Bulletin of the History of Medicine*, *65*, 291-292.

Presidential Commission on the Human Immunodeficiency Virus Epidemic. (1988). *Final Report of the Presidential Commission on the Human Immunodeficiency Virus Epidemic*. Washington, D.C.: Government Printing Office.

Price, M. (1989). *Shattered Mirrors: Our Search for Identity and Community in the AIDS Era*. Cambridge: Harvard University Press.

Project Inform (1989, November). Compound Q—The real story. *PI Perspective*, pp. 1-7.

Project Inform (1991, April). A barrier falls at the FDA. *PI Perspective*, pp. 1-3.

Project Inform (1992, April). AZT in the media. *PI Perspective*, pp. 9-10.

The pros and cons of taking AZT: A roundtable discussion. (1988). In M. Callen (Ed.),

*Surviving and Thriving with AIDS: Collected Wisdom.* New York: PWA Coalition. 2:70-88.

Redfield, R., and D. Burke. (1988, October). HIV Infection: The clinical picture. *Scientific American, 259*(4), 90-99.

Reines, B. (1991). On the locus of medical discovery. *Journal of Medicine and Philosophy, 16*, 183-209.

Research and regulation of HIV drugs. (1988, November). *Exchange*, (9), 1-8.

Robbins, W. (1988, March 16). Doctors urge campaign against AIDS quackery. *New York Times*, p. A21.

Roberts, S. (1990, July). Lab rat: What AIDS researcher Dr. Robert Gallo did in pursuit of the Nobel Prize, and what he didn't do in pursuit of a cure for AIDS. *Spy*, pp. 70-79.

Rogers, D. (1986). Where have we been? Where are we going? *Daedalus, 115*(2), 209-230.

Roman, M. (1988, April). When good scientists turn bad. *Discover*, 50-58.

Root-Bernstein, R. (1993). *Rethinking AIDS: The Tragic Cost of Premature Consensus.* New York: Free Press.

Ruskin, C. (1988). *The Quilt: Stories from the NAMES Project.* New York: Pocket Books.

Russell, S. (1990, June 25). Alternative AIDS symposium sparsely attended. *San Francisco Chronicle*, p. A8.

Saalfield, C. (1990). AIDS videos by, for, and about women. In ACT UP/NY Women and AIDS Book Group (Ed.), *Women, AIDS, and Activism.* Boston: South End. 281-288.

Saalfield, C., and R. Navarro. (1991, May). Not just black and white: AIDS, media, and people of color. *PWA Coalition Newsline*, 15-19.

Salholz, E., et al. (1988, June 6). Acting up to fight AIDS. *Newsweek*, p. 42.

Salholz, E., et al. (1990, March 12). The future of gay America. *Newsweek*, pp. 20-25.

Scarry, E. (1985). *The Body in Pain: The Making and Unmaking of the World.* New York: Oxford University Press.

Schick, R. (1989a, October). Parallel track: Background analysis. *PWA Coalition Newsline*, 60-65.

Schick, R. (1989b, November). The crazy case against AZT. *PWA Coalition Newsline*, 34-40.

Schmeck, H. (1987, March 17). AIDS drug offers hope but cure remains distant. *New York Times*, pp. A1, 16.

Schmeck, H. (1988, June 9). Family tree of AIDS viruses is viewed as 37 to 80 years old. *New York Times*, p. A32.

Schwanberg, S. (1990, Fall). Attitudes toward homosexuality in American health care literature, 1983-1987. *Journal of Homosexuality, 19*, 117-137.

Schwartz, M. (1984). AIDS in the media. In M. Schwartz, *Science in the Streets.* New York: Priority. 87-97.

Sedgwick, E. K. (1990). *Epistemology of the Closet.* Berkeley and Los Angeles: University of California Press.

Seligman, J. (1989, June 12). The mystery of "silent" AIDS infection. *Newsweek*, p. 59.

Serinus, J. (1990/91, December/January). The latest non-toxic natural therapies for AIDS. *PWAlive, 3*(4), 1-13.

Shilts, R. (1989a, May 29). ARC—AIDS resentment complex. *San Francisco Chronicle*, p. A7.

Shilts, R. (1989b, June 9). Montreal meeting debates its goals amid loud protests. *San Francisco Chronicle*, p. A4.

Shilts, R. (1989c, June 26). Politics confused with therapy. *San Francisco Chronicle*, p. A4.

Silver, M. (1988, October 20). FDA offers plan to speed process of drug approval. *Boston Globe*, p. 3.

Smith, D. (1989, July 14). AZT, Acyclovir, and the case for early treatment. *AIDS Treatment News*, pp. 90-93.

Sontag, S. (1989). *AIDS and Its Metaphors*. New York: Farrar, Straus, and Giroux.

Spiers, H. (1989, November/December). AIDS and civil disobedience. *Hastings Center Report*, pp. 34-35.

Thomas, L. (1988). Science and health—possibilities, probabilities, and limitations. *Social Research*, 55(3), 379-395.

Thompson, D. (1990a, January 22). The AIDS political machine. *Time*, pp. 24-25.

Thompson, D. (1990b, July 2). A losing battle with AIDS. *Time*, pp. 42-43.

Thompson, E. P. (1967, December). Time, work-discipline, and industrial capitalism. *Past and Present*, 38, 56-97.

Ticer, S. (1985, December 2). "Fast-buck" artists are making a killing on AIDS. *Business Week*, pp. 85-86.

Todd, A. (1990). Ending the war on disease. *Socialist Review*, 20(3), 99-114.

Treatment Action Group (TAG). (1992, July 20). *AIDS Research at the NIH: A Critical Review. Part I: Summary*. Distributed during the Eighth International Conference on AIDS, Amsterdam.

Treichler, P. A. (1987, Winter). AIDS, homophobia, and biomedical discourse: An epidemic of signification. *October*, 43, 31-70.

Treichler, P. A. (1988). AIDS, gender, and biomedical discourse: Current contests for meaning. In E. Fox and D. Fox (Eds.), *AIDS: The Burdens of History*. Berkeley and Los Angeles: University of California Press. 190-266.

Treichler, P. A. (1989a, October). Seduced and terrorized: AIDS on network television. *Artforum*, 28(2), 147-151.

Treichler, P. A. (1989b). AIDS and HIV infection in the Third World: A First World chronicle. In B. Kruger and P. Mariani (Eds.), *Remaking History*. Discussion of Contemporary Culture, Dia Art Foundation, No. 4. Seattle: Bay Press. 31-86.

Treichler, P. A. (1991). How to have theory in an epidemic: The evolution of AIDS treatment activism. In A. Ross and C. Penley (Eds.), *Technoculture*. Minneapolis: University of Minnesota Press. 57-106.

Treichler, P. A. (1992a). AIDS, HIV, and the cultural construction of reality. In G. Herdt and S. Linderbaum (Eds.), *The Time of AIDS: Social Analysis, Theory, and Method*. Newbury Park, Calif.: Sage. 65-98.

Treichler, P. A. (1992b, January). Beyond *Cosmo*: AIDS, identity, and inscriptions of gender. *Camera Obscura*, no. 28, 21-78,

Treichler, P. A. (1993). AIDS narratives on television: Whose story? In T. Murphy and S. Poirier (Eds.), *Writing AIDS: Gay Literature, Language, and Analysis*. New York: Columbia University Press. 161-199.

Valentine, P. (1988, September 8). Drug researcher pleads guilty to fraud. *Washington Post*, p. A8.

Vollmer, T., et al. (1990, September 20). ACT UP/SF splits in two over consensus, focus. *San Francisco Sentinel*, pp. 1, 4-5.

Waldholz, M. (1989, February 16). Tracking a killer: Merck scientists find a chink in the armor of the AIDS virus. *Wall Street Journal*, pp. A1, A8.

Watney, S. (1987a). *Policing Desire: Pornography, AIDS, and the Media*. Minneapolis: University of Minnesota Press.

Watney, S. (1987b, Winter). The spectacle of AIDS. *October*, 43, 71-86.

Watney, S. (1989). Preface. In S. Watney, *Policing Desire: Pornography, AIDS, and the Media*. 2d ed. Minneapolis: University of Minnesota Press. ix-xiii.

Watney, S. (1990). Photography and AIDS. In C. Squiers (Ed.), *The Critical Image: Essays on Contemporary Photography*. Seattle: Bay Press. 173-192.

Williamson, J. (1989). Every virus tells a story: The meanings of HIV and AIDS. In S. Watney and E. Carter (Eds.), *Taking Liberties: AIDS and Cultural Politics*. London: Serpent's Tail. 69-80.

Yarchoan, R., et al. (1988, October). AIDS therapies. *Scientific American, 259*(4), 110-119.

Young, F. (1988). The FDA's new procedure for the use of investigational drugs in treatment. *Journal of American Medical Association, 259*(15), 2267-2270.

Young, F. (1989). *Public Statement*. National Committee to Review Current Procedures for Approval of New Drugs for Cancer and AIDS.

Young, I. (1988, September 12). Prescription for suicide: Gays, AZT, and mind control. *New York Native*, pp. 18-20.

# Index

ABC news, 15, 16, 18, 20, 29, 137, 138, 139, 140, 141, 142

ACT UP (AIDS Coalition to Unleash Power), 12, 17, 18, 59, 69, 77, 79, 149; and active/passive, 97; and inside/outside, 98; and separationist/assimilationist, 98; negative descriptions of, 96–97; news photographs of, 98, 99; professionalization of, 102; protests, 79, 140, 142; views on alternative treatments, 147; ACT UP/London, 19; ACT UP/New York, 85; ACT UP/San Francisco, 19, 149

Acyclovir, 19, 21

aerosolized pentamidine, 13

AIDS: and subjectivity, 113; and the meaning of "full blown," 39, 82, 139; and tuberculosis, 143; as temporal discourse, 69–88; chronic disease model of, 13–14, 22, 32, 40, 88, 141; critical analyses of media representations of, 108–10; depoliticization of, 30; fatalistic view of, xv, 73, 74, 88; in Asia, 142; meaning of the statistics of, 48–49, 110; normalization of, 13, 44; paradox of curability/incurability of, xi, xv, 32, 36, 37, 68, 70, 89, 91, 94, 102, 130, 133, 135; represented as "diptych," 42–43; tenth anniversary of, 142

AIDS Clinical Trials Group (ACTG), 10

AIDS/HIV education, 34, 36, 61, 62, 63, 64, 65, 66, 67, 70

"AIDS is invariably fatal," xiv, 37–40, 47, 49, 50, 61, 67, 70, 135

"AIDS Kills Fags Dead," 51, 135

*AIDS Quarterly, The,* 34, 36

AIDS treatment activism, xvii, 44, 46, 51, 52, 76, 87, 89; attacks of, 100–101; relation to technomedicine, 54; vs. gay activism, 96, 110

*AIDS Treatment News,* xi

AIDS treatment research: and combination therapy, 18–19, 22, 23, 140; and target drugs, 74; challenge to old standards, xviii; magic-bullet model, xiv, 10, 11, 13, 23, 32; metaphoric descriptions of, 145; rational approach to, 4, 7, 8; vs.

prevention, 101. *See also* clinical drug trials; "curing AIDS"; science

AL-721, 17, 137

alternative treatments, xiv, 10, 36, 56, 58, 67, 94, 140, 147; alternative treatment movement, 56–60; antifraud campaign against alternative treatment movement, 59; history of, 147; underemphasis of, 147

alternative views of AIDS/HIV. See HIV infection

Althusser, Louis, 119, 120

American Council on Science and Health, 30

American Public Health Association, 92

AmFAR (American Foundation for AIDS Research), 17, 85, 138

Amsterdam, xviii, 143

Annas, George, 84

articulation, theory of, xi, xvii, 119, 122; vs. encoding/decoding, 120, 149

AZT (azidothymidine), xiii, 10, 36, 37, 53, 89, 135, 137, 138, 142, 146; ambivalent relation to "curing," 2; approval of, 139; as a success story, 4–8; as orphan drug, 16; as "poison," 24–25, 57; as social and political phenomenon, 2; as tangled narrative, 32–33; "AZT paradigm," 2, 8–14, 28; British study of, 23; budget for, 30; chronological and media history of, 14–28; compared to ddI and ddC, 143; Concorde trial, 22; debate over usefulness of, 2; discovery of, xvii, 2; East Coast vs. West Coast interpretations of, 24; limited distribution of, 25, 27; media representations of, 4–8, 28–33; reactions of blacks and Latinos to, 21; repetitive trials of, 3; usefulness for asymptomatic patients, 141; Veterans Administration study, Round One, 20–21 and Round Two, 22, 23

Barry, David, 16

Barthes, Roland, 69, 70

*Bay Area Reporter,* 52f

Benetton, 45–47

John Nguyet Erni is assistant professor of media and cultural studies in the Department of Communication at the University of New Hampshire, where he teaches courses in popular culture, film theory, gender representations, and AIDS in the media. He has published essays on AIDS and on cultural studies, and is currently working on a book about AIDS and Thailand and the questions of postcolonialism, cultural memory, and sexuality. He is originally from Hong Kong.